TO
PATRICIA
AND TO
ANNA AND MICHAEL

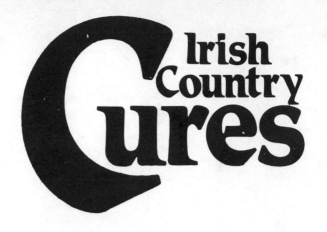

Irish Country Cures

Patrick Logan

Appletree Press

First published in Northern Ireland by
The Appletree Press Limited
7 James Street South
Belfast BT2 8DL
1981

Cased ISBN 0 904651 80 0
Paper ISBN 0 904651 81 9

Published, in Dublin, by the Talbot Press in 1972.

Contents

PART 1

INTERNAL AILMENTS

PART 2

EXTERNAL AILMENTS

PART 3

METHODS OF TREATMENT

PART 4

VETERINARY MEDICINE

Foreword

IN the days of my youth in South Kerry, there lived near us
a man who was known to everybody as 'The Doctor'. At
first I thought that this title was in the nature of a nickname,
but I soon learned that it referred to the powers of healing
which were attributed to the man in question. There were
others too in the parish (all women) who were said to have
curative powers which they had acquired through their
association with the fairies. These were held in a kind of
awe, and many stories were told of their nocturnal travels
with the fairy host.

Then, in the late twenties, I had occasion, while living in
Waterford, to accompany an old neighbour who had a
growth on his lower lip and had travelled all the way from
Kerry to be treated by a woman who lived near the city of
Kilkenny. After giving the old man a cup of tea, the woman
examined the man's lip and, accompanied by her daughter,
went to a room at the lower end of the kitchen; after a
while, they returned, and the woman applied a whitish paste
on a piece of linen (about the size of a florin) to the growth,
warning the man's son, who had also accompanied him, not
to allow his father to tear away the plaster if it pained him
during the night. The woman did not ask for any payment,
but accepted whatever sum was offered to her. The man and
his son returned to Kerry next day, and when I met the old
man two months later, the growth had disappeared, leaving
a small nick on the lip. He died six months later, however,
possibly as a result of the extension of the cancer to other
parts of the body.

Since that time over forty years ago, my work in the folklore field has enlarged considerably my knowledge of folk
medicine. I have come to realise that this subject forms an
integral part of folk culture, not only in Ireland but throughout the world, with basic ideas which are often at variance
with those of the rational world in which we now live.

As late as the seventeenth century, prior to the beginnings
of modern medicine, people the world over could not explain in a rational way the causes of the ailments and diseases from which they occasionally suffered. This led them
to look elsewhere for the sources, and it seemed obvious to
them that the blame for bodily disabilities could be laid
solely on either inimical beings (fairies, spirits, the dead and
such) from an invisible outside world, or else on enemies
who, by means of the evil eye, tongue or heart, could cause
physical harm to those whom they disliked. To cope with
these baneful influences, so-called 'primitive' people had
recourse to either sacrifice (with a placatory purpose) or
magic (the performance of certain acts in a particular way
to secure a definite result). The latter led to the use of verbal
charms, which numbered hundreds, if not thousands, and to
acts of sympathetic magic (such as passing through an open-
ing in the hope of leaving the disease behind). Dr. R. I. Best,
in his bibliographies of early Irish philology and literature,
lists a number of medical tracts and charms, and to these
must be added the very large collections of both charms and
remedies, made mainly in the present century, which are
now in the Folklore Department at University College in
Dublin. As regards charms used for medical purposes, it
must be pointed out that the persons who knew them and the
traditional way in which they should be administered were
very few in any particular area, and these custodians of their
inherited knowledge guarded it jealously.

The therapeutic effectivity of popular medicine cannot be
judged solely from the view-point of modern practice. The
early concepts of disease and the aims of ritual healing were
quite different from those of our own time. A study of folk
medicine must enquire whether it was really effective in its
own environment; whether the folk-healers of earlier generations were able to treat successfully the same ailments as

modern man suffers from and which are now treated in a completely different way; and also, whether folk remedies were especially suitable for certain diseases or groups of diseases. Dr. Logan has, to my mind, successfully faced these problems.

Before commenting on his book in a more detailed way, I should like to refer to the uses to which modern medicine has put some discoveries made—by accident or intuition—by earlier peoples. African medicine-men have for a long time used the bark of a certain type of willow to cure rheumatism with salicyl; the Hottentots knew of aspirin; the natives of the Amazon River basin used cocillana as an effective cough-mixture, and curare, which they applied to arrow-tips to stun their enemies, is now used as an anaesthetic; the Incas have left us cocaine; ephedrine reached the Western World from China; cascara was known to the North American Indians; from the juice of the foxglove was derived digitalin for heart-ailments; and finally, here in Ireland, moulds from which penicillin has been derived were traditionally used for septic wounds. Also, early peoples used compresses, scarification, hot baths (*tithe alluis*), even vaccination; and, if the old saga is to be believed, some kind of trepanning (with a mixture of lime and brain-matter) was tried out on Conchobhar Mac Neasa when his skull had been injured in battle almost two thousand years ago.

The role of healer was a very important one in olden times. Even though some of the herbal and other medications prescribed and used might be lacking in rational effect, nevertheless the manner in which they were applied and used were always of some benefit to the patient. The more complicated the spell or the rite, the more impressed was the sufferer and the relatives. The healer's diagnosis of the ailment and of the cause of it was one of the main parts of his functions. The ceremonial attempt at curing the sick person followed and immediately restored to him the will to recover his health and to live. Just as in modern scientific medicine, the placebo-effect of the medication was to activate the patient's faith. In the olden days, if the ritual curing happened to fail and the patient did not recover, the belief was that a new type of ailment had come into being and the healer was again called in to cope with that. Thus, it may be said that the folk-healer had a social, as well as a medical, function to fulfil—not only those who were ill, but the whole population-group as well, depended on him for advice and help.

I have had the privilege and benefit of reading Dr. Logan's book prior to publication. His work is far from being a casual glance at a very broad, deep and involved subject. As a medical man, he has had a live interest in his subject for over thirty years and has had opportunities of noting folk-remedies from his staff, patients and others from many parts of Ireland. In his comments on various facets of Irish folk medicine, he has shown a most sympathetic approach to the whole problem—an approach, which, I may say, is very welcome and badly needed at the present time when 'folk-lore' is often regarded as of no positive value, as something to be disregarded in serious studies.

I have here a desire to quote a few of his many wise remarks as he goes along: 'Even today the best medicine is reassurance, and the ability to reassure a patient does not always go with a medical degree'; 'almost all physical illnesses —over 80% of them—will get better no matter what treatment is given to them'; 'many of the men and women who practised it (folk-curing) were intelligent and honest and believed in the efficacy of their treatment'; and 'I will be happy if people learn that those who practised folk medicine did good for their patients'. He rightly foresees that as medicine advances and, in some cases, becomes more complicated, it is likely that the practice of folk medicine will decline. That being probably true, we must all owe a debt of gratitude to Dr. Logan for his pioneer work in this hitherto more-or-less neglected field. It is to be hoped too that in the years to come others as able and sympathetic as he will continue the good work, making use of the enormous body of information on this subject which has been recorded in both

Irish and English especially during the past forty years. Not one volume but many will be needed to cover the whole field.

For the present, let us thank Dr. Logan for breaking a road so efficiently through unchartered territory.

SEÁN Ó SÚILLEABHÁIN
(Dept of Folklore, U.C.D.)

Introduction

FOLK medicine, as distinct from official medicine, has always been popular in Ireland, as it has been everywhere else. There are many people who would rather consult an unqualified practitioner than a qualified one and it has been estimated that perhaps one quarter of the medical practice in Ireland today is done by people who are not on the Medical Register. This is not surprising. Even today the best medicine is reassurance and the ability to reassure a patient does not always go with a medical degree.

Nowadays, even with all the wonder drugs, antibiotics, steroids, tranquillisers and the like, the patient's greatest need is still reassurance, and before the days of modern therapy this was even more important. At a time when few drugs had any curative effect, it mattered little if they were prescribed by a qualified doctor or a 'wise woman'; the confidence which went with the treatment made all the difference. Who would say that drinking the water from the well dedicated to the local saint was any less reassuring than an expensive prescription from a consultant physician? It is likely that the use of a charm with its air of mystery and hidden power would be more effective, in the case of some patients, than an official remedy which, after all, does not make any claim to supernatural power.

Now, anyone who treats disease has certain advantages which his patients may not realise. Almost all physical illnesses—over 80% of them—will get better no matter what treatment is given, so it is only common sense on the part of the medical attendant to make sure that he will be given the credit for the favourable result. It must also be realised that more than one third of the people who seek medical advice cannot be found to have any physical cause for their complaints. This is not to imply that these patients are malingering or are dishonest—they are not—but they may be tired or over-worried and they will be greatly helped by being able to tell all their worries to a sympathetic listener. Helped out by a bit of common-sense advice, kindly given, and medicine of some kind, the patient will attribute the relief to the medicine, not to the psychotherapy. Nearly everybody likes to have a few days' rest and the laziest person in the world will believe you if you tell him he needs a rest; it justifies his laziness to himself and is excellent psychotherapy. As a result, he may even believe you when you tell him he is cured.

There is also a large group of diseases, the psychosomatic diseases, in which the physical illness is brought about by some psychological tension. Examples of such conditions are peptic ulcers, asthma, some skin diseases, colitis, many cases of high blood pressure, and thyrotoxicosis. Strictly speaking, these conditions are symptoms of some underlying anxiety, but unfortunately, if not diagnosed and relieved, severe physical disease will often develop which may cause the death of the patient. It is often a very difficult problem to identify the anxiety. In many of the cases, the number of treatments used by official medicine indicates that they are not particularly useful and it has been said that the success or otherwise of the treatment will often depend upon the enthusiasm and faith of the doctor rather than on the direct effect of the drugs he prescribes. Often this is so, and there is no particular reason why an unqualified practitioner who treated asthma should not in some cases get as good results as one with an official qualification.

In the past, qualified physicians were rare and expensive. The result of this was that only the rich consulted them and the great majority of people were treated by the local healer —the person who had the cure of a particular disease or symptom. In the case of a patient with jaundice, for example, a shrewd practitioner would probably be able to decide if the jaundice was due to malignant disease causing obstruction

of the common bile duct and certainly fatal, or the much
more common condition due to infectious hepatitis, in which
the patient recovered. In popular belief, the distinction is
made between the yellow jaundice with a favourable prognosis, and the black jaundice where the prognosis is bad. In
a severe case of hepatitis, where the colouring of the skin is
dark, the medical attendant, qualified or not, will get the
credit for curing the black jaundice.

In some cases the advantage lay with the unqualified practitioner. This was notably so in the case of the hereditary
bone-setters, some of whom still practise in parts of Ireland.
The most notable of such, probably, was the Welsh family
called Thomas. Evan Thomas, an hereditary bone-setter,
realised at the time of the Medical Registration Act in 1858
that his sons must have regular medical qualifications if they
were to continue to practice. The greatest of the sons, Hugh
Owen Thomas, became the founder of the famous Ortho-
paedic school in Liverpool. Before the days of x-rays and
aseptic surgery, a man who had watched his father setting
bones for twenty years was much better able to set a fracture
than the average qualified doctor who had little experience
of this work.

For these reasons it is easy to see why unofficial medicine
flourished. Many of the men and women who practised it
were intelligent and honest and believed in the efficacy of
their treatment, and it must be understood that few of these
people were given any significant amount of money for their
services. True, it was customary to give a small present, but
this was never large and in many cases money was refused.

It is difficult to find the origin of some of these cures.
Many appear to be derived from official medicine. A prescription, for example, of a famous doctor might be written
down and preserved; a number of such prescriptions can be
found in manuscripts of the eighteenth and nineteenth
centuries, and in the prescription books of long-established
chemist shops. The use of the water of a spa well is another
example of official medicine which has become part of folk
medicine and most of the herbal preparations have been at
some time in the Pharmacopoeia. Some of the cures show
brilliant knowledge of human nature: a good example of

such insight is the method of preventing a hare lip. Some are clearly derived from paganism, christianized by means of a few prayers. Some are examples of sympathetic magic, such as the use of yellow flowers to treat jaundice. Some are absurd, some disgusting, and some inexplicable. Some of the more absurd and more disgusting are derived from official medicine. In general the drugs used resemble those found in any mediaeval text book of medicine. A small number will be found useful even today.

Folk medicine provides treatment for all the ordinary and obvious diseases, but it does not deal with certain parts of medicine. Treatments for internal cancers are very rare, and disorders of the central nervous system are almost never treated.

With the development of aseptic surgery, chemotherapy and antibiotics, doctors were inclined to forget that they were dealing with people. There has now been a movement away from this attitude and recently doctors have begun to take more interest in the personality of the patient. Folk curers, not having these material advantages, have not forgotten that they are treating people and therefore they continue to practice successfully because they bring reassurance.

As medicine advances, and in some cases becomes more complicated, it is likely that the practice of folk medicine will decline. Veterinary medicine has become almost entirely official and many of its cures will be forgotten. This is not a complete account of such cures—that would be the work of a lifetime and would require a much longer work.

This book contains the material which I have collected over the past thirty years; most of it was gathered in Counties Leitrim, Cavan and Longford by myself. Most of the remainder has been contributed by friends, the staff and patients of the Dublin Regional Chest Hospital. I was very lucky in this; the members of the staff came from many parts of the country, so that material from nearly every part of Ireland is included. I have written it in the hope that some people will take an interest in folk medicine and record its practices before they are forgotten and I will be happy if people learn that those who practised folk medicine did good for their patients.

I must mention some of the people who helped me: Críostóir O'Muireadhaigh, who told me of the folk medicine of County Westmeath; Sister Margaret Gorman, who told me about County Meath; Miss Margaret Keane, who taught me all I know about the folk medicine of County Clare; Mr. Brendan Garvey, who contributed folk medicine from County Kerry and from County Meath; Miss Catherine Carney, who told me about County Mayo; and Sister Molly Burke, who knew all about the folk medicine of County Wicklow. Two great sources of the folk medicine of Dublin city were Miss Mary Keeley and Mr. Joseph Casey, our visiting dentist. To these, and even more so to those I have not named, I am very grateful.

I must especially mention my friends Tommy Cosgrove of Ballinamore, 'smith and farrier', who told me about the treatment of horses, and Michael Joe Molloy of Milltown, County Galway, who allowed me to consult his notebooks and quote from them. In addition he introduced me to my best contributor of all, Mr. Thomas Acton of Tuam, a well known bonesetter who spoke well for the bonesetters.

My special thanks are due to my friend Miss Christine Finnegan, who did all the hard work reading my crabbed script and typing it, as well as saving me from making many silly mistakes.

Cordoagh
Lucan Road
Chapelizod

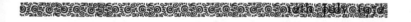

The Practice of Folk Medicine

IN this chapter it is proposed to consider points of folk medicine which are of special interest.

INOCULATION AGAINST SMALL POX

The practice of inoculation against small pox began in western Europe early in the eighteenth century and continued to be a subject of controversy until a much safer practice—vaccination—was introduced by Edward Jenner in 1798. In inoculation, pus from a mild case of small pox was used to infect healthy patients, in the hope that the disease would also be mild and that those inoculated would acquire resistance to the disease. In vaccination the virus of cow pox, closely related to the virus of small pox, is used and as this is a much safer procedure and the degree of immunity conferred is satisfactory the inoculation of small pox was made illegal about the year 1840.

Despite this, a man called Ambrose Donleavy and his son Jimmy Ambrose continued to act as inoculators in County Donegal for a further twenty years at least. As the process was illegal, the inoculator wore a mask so that he could not be identified and those inoculated slept out for some time until their arms had healed. It was believed that the protection against small pox given by the doctors' vaccination only lasted for seven years but that the protection given by the Donleavy's inoculation lasted for life. The Donleavys were presumably members of the famous native Irish medical family, some of whom practised medicine in Counties Donegal, Sligo and Leitrim between the fourteenth and the seventeenth centuries. One of these, probably Paul Ultach who died in 1395, is referred to in a contemporary poem:

> Mac Dhuinnshléibi liaigh na sgol
> Na bia féin is biaidh a bladh.
> (Donleavy Physician of the Schools,
> he will not survive but his fame
> will survive.)

AN FÉAR GORTACH (THE HUNGRY GRASS)

Many people in County Leitrim believe in the hungry grass. The condition is likely to occur after a long day on the mountains rounding up sheep, or more likely shooting. The sufferer feels faint and weak and in severe cases may lose consciousness. After he has rested for some time, usually less than a quarter of an hour, the attack will pass off and he will be able to make his way home. The folk explanation for this dramatic occurrence is that the sufferer happened to walk on hungry grass which caused him to get weak with hunger. There is no doubt that such attacks occur; I have not myself seen one, but many reliable people have told me about them. The attacks may be prevented or cut short by bringing a cake of oaten bread and eating it when the attack begins. The condition appears to be due to a drop in the blood sugar and probably could be treated more quickly with sugar. The reason for the use of the oaten bread is that it is slowly absorbed and has a more prolonged action in raising the blood sugar and keeping it raised.

FOXGLOVE (FAIRY FINGERS)

This striking flower can be found growing everywhere in Ireland. People were slightly afraid of the foxglove and in County Leitrim it was used as a protection against the fairies or against any disease they might cause. Along with barley meal and some other herbs, it was included in a preparation used to treat epilepsy, but I have not been able to learn any more details of the prescription. K'eogh agrees about the epilepsy. He says:

> It is good for any obstruction of the lungs as also for epilepsy.

K'eogh also says that the leaves have an emetic action. They have. On 22nd February 1685 this entry can be found in the Minutes of the Dublin Philosophical Society:

> An account was given how the infusion of foxglove (digitalis flora purpurea), prescribed to a woman above 40 years of age, gave her a violent vomit, without convulsions, which lasted for above two days. She likewise had a palpitation of the heart.

This might be described, in modern language, as 'a near miss', and it would seem that the patient was suffering from digitalis poisoning. It was a pity that the patient was not suffering from congestive heart failure, because if she had the results would have been so dramatic that the honour of the discovery of the uses of digitalis would have gone to the Dublin Philosophical Society.

FEVER

The ordinary infectious fevers no longer occur in Ireland and as a result the folk treatments are not remembered. One method of guarding against fevers was to abstain from meat on the second day of Christmas; this was more effective if the entire family abstained. I once heard of a man who, when told that his sister might have typhoid fever, declared that this was impossible because nobody of their family ever ate meat on the second day of Christmas.

Certain practices to prevent the spread of the infection are still remembered. All the excreta were treated with Jeyes' fluid and then buried in a hole in the ground and when the infection was over a sulphur candle was burned in the room where the patient was nursed.

There is a well-remembered County Kerry pilgrimage which is done in thanksgiving for not getting fever. The pilgrimage consists of a walk from Wether's Well near Tralee to Saint Brigid's Well near Ballyheigue and was established during a fever epidemic in Tralee.

'STUFF A FEVER, STARVE A COLD'

This is an expression which can be heard in most parts of Ireland. It is in a sense the shorthand used in folk medicine for 'he fed fevers'. Many a physician has been given the credit of having cured his fever patients by giving them food when the standard method of treatment was to starve them. But perhaps the man with the best claim to this distinction was Robert Graves of Dublin, who asked that the expression 'he fed fevers' be engraved on his tombstone. It is easy to see how the expression with a slight change in the meaning got itself into Irish folk medicine.

DROPSY

In my native district of County Leitrim, dropsies were treated with Roddy's rope. The belief was that the rope used to hang a man for a crime which he did not commit, if put around the patient, will cure the dropsy, but it was explained that this cure was much more effective in children. My father assured me that during his childhood everyone in the neighbourhood knew that Roddy was innocent, and the rope was kept and used to treat dropsy.

Acute nephritis usually occurs in children or young adults and is a very alarming disease when the face and sometimes the entire body are seen to be swollen. Such cases have quite a good prognosis —more than 90% of them clear up completely and almost all the others improve. This is certainly a shrewd piece of clinical judgement, to distinguish between the prognosis of dropsy in children and in the elderly, when the outlook is quite different.

BURSITIS

Bursae form as protection on bony points of the body which are exposed to continuing pressure, or to minor injuries. Sometimes these bursae (they resemble small sacs) become filled with fluid and may become infected, when they are quite disabling. Examples of these are 'housemaid's knee', got from prolonged kneeling, 'miner's elbow', because miners often lean on an elbow at their work, or 'weaver's bottom', because weavers sit for long hours at the loom.

The treatment of this disabling and painful condition was a poultice of sugar damped and wrapped in strong brown paper. If the infection continued, it would be treated like an ordinary boil, but it was hoped that the sugar and brown paper would help to absorb the fluid in the bursa.

INSOMNIA

As there were no soporifics other than alcohol available generally to folk curers, whiskey was usually given at bedtime. As always, people complained of difficulty in sleeping and a variety of treatments were prescribed, most of which had no soporific effect; yet people were quite certain that they were helpful. I have known a number of people, each of whom had his own method of inducing sleep and could not go to sleep without it. One example was the priest who had a cup of coffee every night at bedtime. Another patient chewed a piece of garlic and still another ate a raw onion. A somewhat unusual method of inducing sleep seemed to work well—the patient slept with his head at the foot of the bed.

CHILD WITH RED CHEEKS

In County Leitrim, people believe that red cheeks in a child is a sign of ill health. I first heard this in answer to a comment on the nice rosy cheeks of a certain child and wondered at the time what it could mean. It may have referred to the hectic red cheeks seen in patients with active tuberculosis and in some cases probably this was so. By the way it was said, the red cheeks appeared to be of some different significance, and I went enquiring about it. All I could learn was 'they don't live long'.

In rare cases, red cheeks may be associated with a condition called polycythaemia (an excessively large number of red blood cells in the circulation). The basic defect is often a congenital disease of the heart and large numbers of red cells are produced to make up for the inefficient action of the deformed heart. This was a shrewd piece of clinical judgement.

'CIS DO CHOIS NÓ SOS DO LÁIMH'

This Irish expression is usually translated 'Stand on your leg but rest your hand', which is not good medical advice about the treatment of an injured foot. It is good advice to immobilise a diseased or injured hand, but it should be equally necessary to immobilise an injured foot. Perhaps the word 'cis' meant restrain, tie up, splint, or bandage, rather than stand on. This would make better medical sense and be more like the advice given in such expressions.

HOSPITAL SUPERSTITIONS

Common practice laid down which relatives should accompany a patient upon admission to hospital. Also in many hospitals it is considered unlucky if a patient goes home on Saturday. 'Saturday flit, short sit' sums it up, but some people consider it most unlucky to move house on Saturday. I am unable to suggest any reason for this belief. It may be derived from the observance of the Jewish Sabbath.

When a patient is being wheeled to the operating theatre, it is customary to move him head first; in coffins, feet go first.

In a ward red and white flowers must never be put in a vase together. People in hospitals say that if this is done one of the patients will die. Perhaps the association of the red with bleeding and the white with anaemia is the explanation. I remember an occasion some years ago when two black crows were seen perched together on the rail of a hospital balcony. Most of the patients did not like it and someone chased them away. The two together were believed to forebode a death.

LEG CRAMPS OCCURRING IN BED

One lady who suffered severely from recurring cramps in the muscles of her legs had consulted many doctors and had had the condition very thoroughly investigated. Many official forms of treatment had been used but the cramps persisted until she consulted a folk curer. The folk curer told her to get a muslin bag and fill it with an assortment of corks and the bag of corks must be put in her bed. She did this and now for many years she has not had any cramps.

RABIES

It is more than a lifetime since a case of hydrophobia was reported in this country, but people still speak of the bite of a mad dog and any dog bite is treated very seriously. The fear of the disease is very old in Ireland and may be illustrated by this quotation from a fifteenth century book of the Irish laws:

There is no benefit in proclaiming it (the dog) unless it
be killed, nor though it be killed unless it be burned,
nor though it be burned unless the ashes be cast into
a stream.

This killing, burning and casting into a stream is very
ancient magic. There are examples of casting things into
water in Anglo-Saxon magic to clean them or cure them or
take away the evil. There is another reference in the Irish
laws which ordered that a house in which an injured man
was treated and nursed should have a stream of water running through the middle of the floor.

Jonah Barrington in his Recollections mentions a case
when a man who was believed to be suffering from hydrophobia was smothered between two feather ticks. This story
was told with Barrington's usual trimmings about the peasan-
try and I did not believe it until my father showed me a man
whose grandfather had been smothered in a similar way
because he had hydrophobia. My father and other men of his
generation in County Leitrim did not consider this treatment unfair: the danger justified it and the patient was going
to die anyway.

A man called MacGovern, living in Glangevlin in County
Cavan, where almost everyone is called MacGovern, was
famous as a curer of hydrophobia. This man is long dead
and I have been unable to learn exactly what was used, but
barley meal and crowfoot leaves were used, as well as a hair
of the dog that bit the patient. People were rather reluctant
to speak about rabies and it was also thought to be unlucky
for the curer. With such a general fear, it was almost routine
that the dog be killed. The success of MacGovern's cure seems
to be due to the fact that hydrophobia was a very rare disease and dog bites were common. Surely not one in a hundred
dog bites was followed by hydrophobia, but everyone bitten
in the neighbourhood of Glangevlin was treated with the
cure and every biting dog killed.

TETANUS

I have a very clear memory of seeing a pig which was
reputed to have died of lock-jaw. I do not know if the diag-

nosis was correct, or even if pigs suffer from lock-jaw, but people thought that they did. There is a belief that a cut in the fleshy web between the thumb and first finger may cause tetanus. This, of course, is no more true than of any other cut and I have often wondered why this belief arose. As tetanus is a disease of country people, people who work on the land with their hands, injuries to the hands are common and there are often cracks in the hard skin. Certainly, a hand injury is much more likely to be contaminated with tetanus germs than any other injury.

AN FIOLÚN

My friend Father Patrick O'Sullivan, O.F.M., told me of a treatment for fiolún of which he had heard in the Connemara Gaeltacht. When asked what fiolún was, the healer said it was 'lot'. Lot means harm or injury. The word fiolún is used in the Irish annals for the enlarged and often suppurating glands which occurred in some cases of plague. Perhaps in this case fiolún meant some form of chronic ulcer. In carrying out the treatment it was necessary that the patient be completely buried in the earth. When asked about the danger of smothering the patient, the healer explained that the patient only remained covered for a moment.

This is an example of pagan magic in which the disease is transferred to the earth, which is the great healer and purifier. Such transference cures are found in folk medicine everywhere.

MIDWIFERY

One of the oldest investigations in human medicine must be the tests to determine the sex of an unborn child. Many such tests can be found scattered in Irish manuscripts, and here are two of them taken from a manuscript, O'Curry No. 8, in the Library of Saint Patrick's College, Maynooth. This is a seventeenth century manuscript in Latin and Irish of the Aphorisms of Hippocrates. Some notes in English were probably written in this manuscript during the early years of the eighteenth century. One note reads:

> To know whether a woman be with childe with a male
> or female. If (the) first the complexion will be a little bit

altered, the right breast round and firm, the nipple hard and red.

The other test was:

You make a cake with woman's milk, when she is with child, and when baking it continues hard and firm, it denotes she goes with a boy.

A twentieth century method of determining the sex of an unborn baby is attributed to a well known Dublin obstetrician. When one of his patients asked him whether she was going to have a boy or a girl, he said whichever one he thought she would prefer. However, if he indicated that he thought the baby would be a boy, he was careful to write on the patient's chart that he thought she would have a girl. Then he could say to the patient after the delivery: 'Now, didn't I tell you that you would have a girl?' and when the patient said: 'No, you told me the baby would be a boy', the chart was produced to show that she was mistaken.

In County Longford there was an interesting method of dealing with any difficulty which might arise during labour. If, for example, the labour was unduly prolonged, the anxious husband was called and told about the problem. It was then his duty to find the heaviest flagstone he could and carry it around the house; the heavier the stone, the better. When he had completed the job, and returned to report, he might be sent off and told to do it again and look for a heavier stone. If a modern psychologist ever heard of this practice, he might say it was a good way of involving the father in the drama of childbirth. I don't know if we peasant Irish ever thought of it like that, but it was a very good method of getting him out of the way when he would very likely be a nuisance.

Another method to speed up labour may have been used in County Longford. If the patient has long hair, a ball is made of this and an attendant tries to shove it down her throat. The violent efforts of the patient to get rid of it to avoid choking would help to expel the foetus.

There are all sorts of stories about the luck of a child born with a caul. This is one of the membranes which is on rare occasions found around the child when it is delivered. In such a case, the caul is preserved by the mother and as long as she keeps it the child will not be drowned. The mother may also keep it and give away small pieces to protect sailors, fishermen, drivers and travellers in general. Some people believe that an individual born with a caul is very lucky, and I have heard a story about people who wished to share Sweepstake tickets with such a person.

There are many methods of ensuring an easy labour. One certain method is for the mother to eat fish brains during pregnancy. I once heard a story about people who were surprised in a church while trying to take a piece of skin from a dead body which was to be used to help a woman in labour. This seemed like a tall story, but K'eogh has a horror-chapter in his book Zoologia Medicinalis Hibernica called 'The Medicinal Virtues of the Parts Extracted from human bodies'. The powers and virtues of the parts and products of homa vivens and homo mortuus are even more absurd and disgusting than the rest of the book. One of the less disgusting recommendations reads: 'The skin worn about the belly facilitates labour and cures hysterical disorders.'

HARE LIP

Years ago when people used greyhounds to hunt hares, the hunter, even before he picked up the hare to carry it home, must be sure to pull out the tail (scut) of the animal. This practice was observed in many parts of Ireland, but only in Country Leitrim could I learn why it was done. If the hunter did not do it and on his way home he met a pregnant woman her baby might be born with a hare lip. It is easy to laugh this off as an example of childish superstition, but that is to take a very superficial view of the problem. Parents are, naturally, very anxious about any congenital deformity in their children and wish to know why this should have happened. Perhaps both have secret guilt feelings about it and a hare lip is a very noticeable deformity. If it can be attributed to something like meeting a man carrying a hare from which the scut has not been removed, then everybody is greatly relieved and the parents' feeling of responsibility is so much the less. Even for the mother to see a hare running is not without danger to the unborn child.

A similar belief, which is also found in Counties Cavan and Leitrim, is that a pregnant woman should not go to a funeral and it is even dangerous if she happens to meet one on the road. Should either of these things happen, the baby may be still-born or the woman may have a miscarriage. Recently I have heard of a lady who had a miscarriage and this was attributed to the fact that she had gone to the funeral of her mother-in-law. Again it is a case of being able to escape from the responsibility.

UMBILICAL HERNIA IN AN INFANT

When this is seen in a newborn baby it can often be treated efficiently and simply. In the days before aseptic midwifery, it may have been more common, because the stump of the umbilical cord was likely to be infected. The hernia was treated by wrapping a penny (an old penny) in cloth and putting it over the hernial sac. This was covered with a pad and firm bandage. To make sure that the penny remained in the correct position, a small many-tailed bandage could be used. When some years ago a Jubilee Nurse was first appointed to a County Longford parish, the Parish Priest spoke about it in his sermon, Having advised his flock to avail themselves of her help, he ended:

> I do not wish to say anything against the handy women. They were very good, I was brought into the world myself by a handy woman, Lord have mercy on her, and you could hang your hat on my navel to this day.

CLUB-FOOT

In milder cases of club foot early treatment is often simple and efficient. The foot is turned into the correct position. Then a flat board, well padded with wool, is placed along the outside of the baby's foot which is bandaged to it.

There is a well dedicated to Saint Bernard near to Abbey Knock Moy in County Galway. This well is visited by newly married women to ensure that they will become pregnant. The story is told of an elderly farmer in north Galway who got married and was very anxious to have a son. He went on pilgrimage to Knock to pray for a son but his wife had a daughter. He then went on the pilgrimage to Croagh Patrick and again his wife had a daughter. Some of the neighbours advised him to visit Saint Bernard's well and he finally decided to go. When his wife had a third daughter he was heard to say: Ach, these saints don't understand, and he 'let down his feathers and died'.

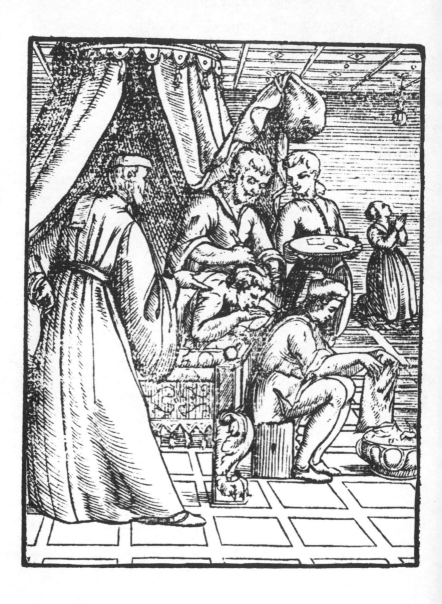

Part 1

Internal Ailments

CHAPTER I

The Chest

COUGH and spit are the chief characteristics of diseases of the chest and the number of cough mixtures still in use is evidence that people are afraid of a cough which continues for any length of time. Tuberculosis of the lungs has now become a rare disease, but for long it was a major problem in Ireland. Similarly bronchitis—both acute and chronic—and pneumonia were very important diseases for which, until thirty years ago, official medicine had no specific treatment. The folk cures for these illnesses are mainly derived from official medicine.

TUBERCULOSIS OF THE LUNGS

The treatment of this condition has now ceased to be part of Irish folk medicine. A little more than twenty years ago, however, the patients in an Irish sanatorium used to go regularly to a folk curer who lived about ten miles away. The visits were well organised and each group went in its turn. When some changes were made in the staff of the institution and these visits were no longer possible, two patients who had not been to the curer were very disappointed. In order to make up for this, their fellow patients subscribed enough money to send them to Lourdes.

About the same time, the Minister for Health was asked in the Dáil if he would make a widely advertised cure for tuberculosis available to Irish patients.

The official name of a well-known Irish sanatorium was 'The Royal National Hospital for Consumption in Ireland', but the postal address was 'The Anchor Hotel', Newcastle,

County Wicklow. It was socially quite acceptable to stay at a hotel while recovering from an illness—it might even be a spa—but many people were very reluctant to admit that they had a relative being treated in a tuberculosis hospital, even The Royal National Hospital for Consumption in Ireland.

Formerly, a popular treatment for tuberculosis was to drink a cupful of linseed oil daily. Similarly, a cough mixture made of flax seed boiled in water to form a thin paste was used. This was made less nauseous by adding sugar and honey, but even so it was not easy to take. The use of linseed in treatment of chest diseases is part of mediaeval medicine. Marryat (1764) advised: 'infusion of linseed or decoction of bran', as part of his treatment for tuberculosis, and K'eogh wrote about linseed:

> Mixt with honey and taken as an electuary it is a great pulmonic, good against all disorders of the lungs.

I have heard of two Dublin cures for tuberculosis. One is that the patient must drink four teaspoonfuls of paraffin oil daily. The other treatment is a sandwich of bread and butter with a filling of fresh dandelion leaves. Another cure, this time from County Leitrim, consisted of two raw eggs beaten up with sugar and a little whiskey. The raw eggs were given routinely to sanatorium patients and I know one man who, as a sanatorium patient in 1935, made himself sick eating beaten up raw eggs.

Garlic is of course a most popular medicine for curing lung diseases in general and tuberculosis in particular. It was grown in many Irish gardens to be used both for its flavour and as a medicine. The cloves were boiled, macerated in the water, and strained. Honey was added to the liquid, which was then used as a cough medicine. K'eogh gives almost the same prescription:

> Take a handful of it (Garlick) and boil it in two quarts of spring water to the consumption of a quart. Then strain it and put a quart of honey to it, of which make a syrup. Take a spoonful of this at a time and it will infallibly cure any cough, asthma, shortness of breath, etc.

One other treatment may be mentioned. Carrigeen to

which nasturtium seeds have been added is boiled and drunk.
In one Irish sanatorium, rows of pine trees have been
planted in the grounds. In the opinion of the lady who did
excellent work in helping to found the institution, the smell
of the pine could cure tuberculosis, so she had the trees
planted.

Goats have a high resistance to tuberculosis and formerly it
was often advised to drink goat's milk. The Kerry breed of
cattle also has a high resistance and the milk of the little
black cows was also advised.

I have also been told seriously that in order to be cured of
tuberculosis one must sleep with a buck goat for six weeks!

Here is an official cough mixture which can be found in
an Irish nineteenth century manuscript, 23.G.41 in the Royal
Irish Academy. The entry is headed:

> Cure for cough, Dr. O'Loughlin's Recipi:
> Take the yolk of a new laid egg, and six spoonfuls of
> Red Rose water and beat well together, and make each
> time sweet with white sugar candy, and drink six nights
> going to bed.

The Doctor O'Loughlin mentioned probably was Brian
O'Lochlainn, M.D., who died on 18th September 1734. This
man appears to have studied in Paris and returned to his
native County Clare to practice medicine.

There were many euphemisms used in common speech
when one did not like to say 'tuberculosis' or, even worse,
'consumption'. One might say: 'ah, the poor girl is not
strong'. For people who were 'not strong', calf's foot jelly was
the treatment of choice. I remember an old lady who used
to get the feet of cattle and boil them to make the jelly. As
she made it, the stuff was a light grey and not very attractive
looking, but a commercial preparation, clear, bright and
attractive, was quite popular.

People in Ireland greatly feared what they called 'a summer
cold'. It was well recognised that a 'cold' which came on
during the summer and persisted might be a very serious
illness and one is often told by a patient with tuberculosis
that his disease began with a summer cold. Tuberculosis
might manifest itself as fluid on the chest and this also was

greatly feared. It was widely believed that, in very hot weather, one should not over-exert oneself in the sun, and if for some reason one did so it was particularly dangerous to sit on wet grass or worse to sit on a cold stone. There is a very good foundation for this belief. The danger of re-activating tuberculosis by sitting in the hot sun is well recognised and certainly pleural effusions most often occur during hot weather.

BRONCHITIS IN CHILDREN

A child with an acute attack of bronchitis may be quite ill, but, whether ill or not, his parents will be very worried about him. For the mild bronchitic condition associated with the pain and discomfort of teething, it is advised that he be taken to where the road is being tarred so that he can smell the tar. This is the usual Dublin method of treating whooping cough.

For a child who is 'caught' on the chest, a preparation of garlic is used. In this case the leaves and cloves of the garlic are all chopped very fine, wrapped in brown paper and applied to the chest. I have cut up garlic as though to prepare this plaster and the smell of the garlic is very strong and it is probable that whatever action the plaster may have is due to the smell. In this, it resembles some well known patent medicines which may be rubbed on the chest and which have pleasant medicinal smells.

Ivy leaves may be chewed and the juice swallowed to 'clear' the chest. K'eogh says:

> The juice of the leaves cures wounds, ulcers, burns, scalds, snuffed into the nose, purges the head of slimy viscid cold humours.

A similar treatment is to chew, suck and swallow the juice of dandelion leaves.

PNEUMONIA

Until the introduction of the sulphonamide drugs, and later the antibiotics, pneumonia was a very grave illness. At that time the treatment was designed to help the patient overcome the disease by his own natural powers. One of the most important forms of treatment was the use of poultices and other such applications to the chest, which probably added to the patient's comfort. One of these which was used in Dublin consisted of rubbing a big stick of tallow made up in the shape of a thick old-fashioned candle all over the chest. When this had been done, the chest was covered with strong black paper and then covered with a woollen cardigan to keep it in place. The paper might also be sewn on to an inside garment. The rubbing with the tallow must be repeated daily for nine days or until the crisis occurs.

This use of paper is one of a number of 'Papers' which were part of official medicine until a few years ago. They were usually counter-irritants and designed to relieve pain. Here is another one which also became a folk treatment for pneumonia: mustard powder was wetted and mixed with honey and spread on brown paper which was then applied to the chest to relieve pain. It might, of course, be used to relieve pain in any other part of the body and is probably derived from the official Charta Sinapis. Officially this was prepared by smearing on one ounce of mustard powder mixed in two ounces of Gutta Percha. The instruction read:

It should be dipped in tepid water before use.

The most usual poultices were of linseed meal and kaolin. These ceased to be used when the antibiotics became available to treat pneumonia. They have now been given up as folk remedies, largely because they are no longer necessary.

There is one poultice for the chest which appears to be a genuine folk remedy. Wool from a black sheep is taken and arranged to fit the chest. Onions are fried in grease and spread on the wool, which is then applied. Sometimes mustard is added to the preparation and it is stuck on with white of egg. The point about the colour of the wool is probably very old. There are examples rather like this in Anglo-Saxon folklore. The milk or butter of a cow of one colour is used in many Anglo-Saxon cures. It is also found in old Irish. Originally the idea of one colour may have been associated with purity.

A GREEN CHRISTMAS MAKES A FAT CHURCHYARD

In order to grasp the significance of this saying, one must

know something about the housing conditions in Ireland
during the nineteenth century or earlier. If the weather was
cold it was dry and, as people had plenty of turf and used it
in plenty, they were able to keep warm. During a mild wet
winter conditions were very different. Clothes and beds were
damp and people suffered from chest infections. This was
much more likely in elderly people. They went to damp
beds and curled up to keep warm and what was originally
a mild chest infection developed into congestion of the bases
of the lungs and pneumonia. There was not often a fireplace
in a bedroom, and if there was one the chimney was probably stuffed. Such conditions were not peculiar to Ireland;
they existed everywhere during cold damp weather. Such
a mild, creeping pneumonia was described by Osler as 'the
natural end of old people'.

ASTHMA IN CHILDREN

This is, to a great extent, a psychosomatic disorder and,
as might be expected, there are many forms of treatment
for it. A standard one was made with the leaves of colt's-foot
boiled in milk and the entire preparation was eaten. Colt's-
foot is a very old preparation and K'eogh was enthusiastic
about its virtues. He wrote:

> It is a very great pectoral herb, good for all diseases of
> the lungs, coughs, consumptions, etc.

Sundew is also used to treat asthma. In this case the leaves
are chopped up fine and the juice squeezed out. The juice
is bottled and, when needed, a few drops are added to a
tablespoonful of honey. This is a surprising preparation because the leaves of the sundew applied as a poultice are a
strong counter-irritant and this may have been its principal
use in chest diseases.

Two other methods of treating asthma in children may be
mentioned. In one case a saucer containing vinegar was placed
on a table beside the child's bed and the fumes from it
relieved the attacks during the night. In the other chopped
onions were boiled in milk and given to the child. I understand that this would work very well if the patient could
be persuaded to take it.

INFLUENZA

There were two severe epidemics of influenza in this country, one about the year 1884 and the other in 1918. These were remembered in my youth and people were inclined to say 'the flu, God help us'. As a result, any disease which was called 'the flu' was treated seriously. One method was to give the patient as much gruel as he could be persuaded to take. A pleasant form of treatment was beef tea. I remember well being given it and the way I finished it all must have been very good for my mother. Another method of treatment was stout mulled with a red hot poker. The most popular form of treatment was *poitín* (illicit whiskey) sweetened with honey.

After such enjoyable forms of treatment, eating boiled flax seed is not pleasant. Unfortunately, all the authorities agreed that it was a sovereign remedy so it had to be taken. This is what Whitla wrote about it:

> Flax seed contains a mucilaginous principle which it yields to boiling water, and which acts as a soothing demulcent when it comes in contact with the gastrointestinal mucous membrane. . . . It has reputed expectorant qualities.

THE COMMON COLD

All the usual mixtures, already mentioned, were used to treat colds; egg white; honey; linseed oil; sugar and mulled stout, etc. One rather elaborate mixture contained honey to which lemon juice had been added and all cooked into a thick paste with flour. If someone was caught out in cold rain or, worse, in fog, a glass of hot milk well laced with rum was given. A tickling cough in the throat might be relieved by a small pat of butter which had been rolled in sugar. The Dublin mixture was equal parts of porter and milk, sweetened with sugar.

CHAPTER II

The Heart

THERE are few Irish folk remedies for diseases of the heart. This is not surprising. There was only one efficient heart drug—foxglove leaves—available to official medicine during the nineteenth century and, although this was derived from an English folk remedy for dropsy, it does not appear to have been so used in Ireland. True, foxglove was used in Irish folk medicine, but not for any symptom which might be associated with heart disease.

There is one notable method of investigating and treating diseases of the heart which is probably still being used in many parts of Ireland. It is well known that a pain in the chest may be caused by serious heart disease. This has been known to official medicine since the middle of the eighteenth century (Heberden's Angina Pectoris), but the cause of the pain was not known and there was no clear-cut line of treatment and no great results from any treatment. In Irish folk medicine, angina pectoris might be translated *croí-chrá* (heart pain) or *feochair chroí,* which means much the same.

In such circumstances it might be expected that folk medicine would evolve a method of diagnosis, prognosis and treatment for the *croí-chrá,* and it did so. As in the case of skin cancer, the patient, when he suffered an attack of chest pain, first consulted a doctor to have the diagnosis of heart disease confirmed. The doctor could not always be sure of the cause of the pain, so he issued a general warning. The sufferer, or his friends, then sought the aid of the person who treated the heart pain.

There were some variations in the ritual of the treatment,

but the general idea was much the same as this one used in County Leitrim: it was necessary that the patient be put to bed and that he remain there for the necessary nine, or ten, days. The person making the cure filled an egg cup with oat meal and covered the mouth of the egg cup with a muslin cloth. The egg cup was then put—mouth downwards—on the site of the chest pain and expertly bandaged in position, where it must remain undisturbed for the nine days. When the bandages were removed by the folk curer he was able, by examining the amount of meal in the egg-cup, to decide what the prognosis for the patient was likely to be. If the amount of meal had not grown less, it might be because the heart was healthy and did not need any treatment. It might also be taken to mean that the meal was not able to get in to treat the diseased heart. If a considerable amount of the meal had gone, this meant that it had been used up in treating the sick heart, which must therefore have been severely diseased. With all these possible choices, the prognosis depended on the acumen of the person making the cure and, as a preliminary, it was a safe practice to keep the patient in bed for nine days. At the end of that time it might be clear that the patient was well and a good prognosis could be given. If, on the other hand, the patient was still ill, a properly guarded prognosis could be given by examining the meal.

Some variations in the ritual may be noted. A glass or a cup may be used to hold the meal. The dressing may be taken down and the meal examined on the third, sixth, and ninth days. This gave the person making the cure a reason to visit and examine the patient. Sometimes a cake was made of the meal at each visit and eaten by the patient and fresh meal was put in the glass.

This treatment, which began as a treatment for chest pain which might be due to the blocking of an artery of the heart muscle, or to insufficient oxygen reaching the muscle for any reason, began to be used in other diseased conditions of the heart. For this reason it was less successful as a method of prognosis and it is now used less than in former years.

The *feochair chroí* is treated by a different method in Donegal. The person making the cure uses a piece of silk ribbon about a yard long. Two pieces of thread of the same length as the ribbon are placed one on each side of it and all three are then rolled up together. The curer then takes the roll in his right hand and makes the Sign of the Cross on the front of the chest and behind it with the roll. When the ribbon is unrolled, the threads will be found to be reversed if the prognosis is good. This cure is hereditary and must be transmitted from a man to a woman, who in turn gives it to a man.

Even today, with accurate and sophisticated methods of investigation, it is often difficult to give an accurate prognosis in the case of a patient suffering from chest pain. Some of the people who made these cures had become quite skilful and were sometimes able to give an accurate opinion. I have heard of one patient who had suffered from congestive heart failure for a number of years who had this cure made. The healer realised that the outlook was poor and was able to tell the patient's relatives.

The dropsy, associated with congestive heart failure, is a very noticeable feature, but the outlook was, until recently, so poor that there were almost no folk remedies for it. One such case which I studied nearly twenty-five years ago is of some interest. The patient, a lady, had her oedema treated by the official medical remedies of the seventeenth century. This consisted of reducing her intake of fluids and giving her what official medicine of the seventeenth century called cholagogues, as well as emetics and sweating. The purgatives given were croton oil, large doses of salts, jalap and scamony. The emetic given was mustard and, to add to her discomfort, she was sweated with blankets and hot water bottles during a hot summer.

CHAPTER III

The Gastro-Intestinal Tract

INDIGESTION

THIS is a very vague word and can be used for many
conditions. Its importance can be judged by the number of
patent medicines which claim to cure it—whatever it is.
In a general way it may be considered as a condition of
abdominal discomfort, often associated with the taking of
certain foods and often made worse by anxiety or worry.
The former Professor of Gastro-Enterology at the Mayo
Clinic, W. C. Alvarez, wrote a brilliant book on the condition which he called 'Nervousness, Indigestion and Pain'.
In Irish folk medicine there is a condition called displacement of the cléithín or in other parts of the country it is
said that the spoon of the chest is down. The spoon of the
chest (cléithín) was the small piece of cartilage at the lower
end of the breast bone, which if pressed upon caused a certain amount of vague discomfort. It was generally believed
that if this cartilage was displaced it caused indigestion.

When a patient complained of indigestion and consulted
the healer, he examined the cartilage and, if he found that
it had been displaced, he undertook to replace it. The basic
method was to heat a glass which was then pressed to the
skin over the cartilage. As the patient watched, he could see
the sucking effect on the skin as the air in the glass cooled.
A more elaborate ritual required that a cake of oatmeal
bread, not baked, be placed over the area and a lighted
candle stuck in the dough. The curer warmed the glass with
the candle and then applied it to the skin. Perhaps the cake
of oatmeal was used to make an airtight seal around the

mouth of the glass. I did not learn if any prayers were said in making this cure, but I did hear of one lady in County Galway who had quite a reputation for her skill in replacing the cléithín. She gave up the practice when two or three members of her family died. It was sometimes necessary to repeat the ritual a few times before the improvement was satisfactory.

Any relief of the indigestion which followed this treatment was due to good psychotherapy. The person performing the cure would probably be well able to estimate what the result was likely to be, so he could give an accurate prognosis.

WIND IN THE STOMACH

This is usually due to the patient's habit of swallowing air. He becomes very conscious of his swollen belly and is able to relieve it by belching—which he can do—loudly and clearly. One method of treating this condition is to give the patient half a pint of milk to which four teaspoonsful of fine soot have been added. This is a folk version of an official treatment: 'for flatulent conditions of the stomach and intestines', when the carbon was believed to absorb the stomach gases. This mixture of milk and soot is also used to relieve the crampy abdominal pains which are associated with food poisoning or other types of irritation of the gut.

DIARRHOEA

Diarrhoea is an obvious and rather embarrassing symptom. It may be due to a number of conditions and, as the folk curers knew this, they treated it with a certain amount of caution. The most likely cause in nineteenth century Ireland was probably food poisoning and this could be helped in most cases. A pint of water was used to dissolve two teaspoonsful of salt and to this the white of two eggs beaten stiff was added. The patient was given four ounces of this mixture and if he had not vomited it within a quarter of an hour he was given the rest. This treatment may be repeated four times daily.

In a severe case the mixture of salt and water would be very useful in replacing the lost water and salt, and the egg white would provide some protein of high quality for the patient in a very digestible form.

Another method of treating diarrhoea was to use the meacan buí an tsléibhe (the mountain spurge) which is said to be an infallible cure. K'eogh says about the spurges:

> They are all very great cathartics, they purge viscous phlegm and choleric humours.

In any case, these virtues are not important because all the patient had to do was gather a few of the roots and sit on them.

Another method is to boil the bark of the barberry bush and drink the liquid. As well as diarrhoea, this is reputed to cure liver diseases. K'eogh has this to say about it:

> The inner bark (which is of a deep yellow colour) is accounted a specific against the yellow jaundice. The fruit is styptic therefore good against all kinds of fluxes.

Another form of treatment is boiled blackberry roots. Here K'eogh reported:

> The roots are good against the stone and provoke urine. . . . The decoction of them (the young buds) stop the flux of the belly . . . and all fluxes of blood.

It would appear that someone got his authorities mixed up. However, it could not make any significant difference to the patient whether a decoction of the roots or of the young buds was given him: the water in which the stuff was boiled would be of some benefit.

PEPTIC ULCER

Irish folk medicine knew nothing about peptic ulcers, but people were very much aware of what they called 'a bad stomach'. Everybody knew that baking soda would relieve pain after taking food, but there was a widespread fear of it. People said that it would take the lining off the stomach and I have heard the expression 'he was always taking baking soda' used about a man who ultimately developed cancer of the stomach. There was no definite diet prescribed for these cases. Milk and cream and water were advised, but I knew one man who said he cured his 'bad stomach' with a diet of raw eggs beaten up in milk and cream crackers.

Some things were considered very bad. One of these was bread of which only one side was toasted. Others were goose, duck, and salt beef. Another was tea without milk or sugar. Treacle was considered very good and also soup. One old Dublin treatment for a bad stomach is of interest. A dried fig was broken up and left soaking in olive oil overnight. The patient took the fig and the oil fasting in the morning.

PILES

There are innumerable forms of treatment for piles, most of which could not possibly have any effect on the condition. The wild buttercup is used to make two cures. In one case the roots, ground up, are boiled with lard and made into an ointment. Another method advises that the leaves be boiled, two handfuls in a pint of water. The patient is told to drink the water.

A notably useless method of treatment is to set fire to a piece of tarred rope. This is placed in a metal bucket and the sufferer squats over the bucket and the smoke cures the piles.

A more realistic form of treatment is a poultice of boiled onions. This, I have been assured, gives considerable relief and K'eogh says:

> They open the piles being externally applied with oil and vinegar.

It is likely that the vinegar would be quite painful.

Flowers of sulphur has a reputation for the treatment of piles. It was advised by a well known Irish physician, Doctor Neligan, but its use appears to be much older. The only preparation which I have found contained flowers of sulphur one ounce, and linseed oil half a pint. A tablespoonful was taken twice daily.

WORMS

I have heard of few folk cures for intestinal worms, although there were many. Children were given a half pint of lime water daily for a week. Another treatment was the boiled roots of nettles. This would probably be a strong purgative. In County Leitrim I heard of a cure for worms which was attributed to a Leitrim Franciscan friar, Father Gregory Dunne. A piece of paper on which the words

et verbum carum factum est

were written was used to make the Sign of the Cross over water which was then given to the child to drink.

When I was young, people believed that if orange pips were swallowed they might cause appendicitis. This was taken over from a famous mistake. When appendectomy became a popular operation small concretions closely resembling orange pips were sometimes found in the appendix. When, some time later, these were examined more thoroughly they were found to be faecaliths.

CHAPTER IV

The Urinary Tract

SOME charms against urinary disease (an galar fuail) have been found in old Irish manuscripts. An galar fuail is mentioned as a cause of death on a number of occasions in the Irish annals and may have been due to stones in the kidneys or in the bladder. It would seem more likely, however, that the condition meant was obstruction of the neck of the bladder by an enlarged prostate gland.

One of the charms reads:

> A charm against urinary disease. 'I save myself from this disease of the urine . . . save us cunning birds, bird flocks of witches save us.' This is always put in the place in which thou makest thy urine.

I do not understand this completely, but it seems that the patient repeated the invocation. It may have been written down and placed in the urinal. Certainly it shows no Christian influence.

Another charm against urinary disease has been found in the Stowe Missal. The words of this charm which are to be repeated by the person performing the cure, in the hearing of the patient, or perhaps by the patient himself are:

> Fuil fuiles camul lind lindas gaine rath reththe srothe telc tuse lotar taora mucca inanais bethade nethur siul narosiul na rosuil. Taber no fuil in ait oneitt agus toslane. Roticca ic slane.

Whitley Stokes translated the last ten words:

Put thy urine in . . . thy . . . and thy health. May a cure of health heal thee.

The first twenty words are Irish, but it is not possible to translate them or to get any meaning from them. It has been suggested that such incomprehensible words are survivals of a forgotten language and one example of it can be found in this work. In the case of this charm, this does not appear to be so. It is more likely that the incomprehensible words are used to impress the patient who was probably made to repeat them. The fact that the patient was able to understand the last few words was very good psychology and he would be pleased and flattered. In a work on Anglo-Saxon medicine and magic by Bonser a similar type of charm is quoted, which is also a mixture of words which the patient understands and words which he cannot understand.

In modern Irish folk medicine there are not many forms of treatment for urinary diseases still in use. Of the group of diseases the two most important are kidney stones and difficulty in passing water due to enlargement of the gland at the neck of the bladder. In the days before official medicine could deal efficiently with these conditions, folk medicine could do as much, or as little, so it was up to the patient to have the college doctor or the folk healer. Sometimes surgeons were prepared to open the bladder and remove a stone, but this was an operation which few had the physical courage to undergo. It will be found that the folk remedies still remembered are derived from the official medicine of a few hundred years ago and folk medicine does not appear to have been able to improve on them.

One form of treatment still not forgotten is the use of parsley for urinary diseases. I was unable to find out exactly how it was prepared but one of my informants said that the roots were boiled, he thought. However, K'eogh was of help. He had this to say about the virtues of parsley:

A Decoction of the Roots and Seed, drank, opens obstructions of the Liver, Kidneys and all the Internal Parts. It Provoketh urine and expelleth the stone and gravel.

Dandelion is also used to treat diseases of the urinary tract.

In this case both the leaves and the roots are used. The leaves are brewed to make what is called dandelion tea to increase the output of urine. K'eogh agrees with this and says among many other virtues that it:

Cleans the reins (kidneys) and bladder.

I have also heard that the entire plant, roots and all, should be boiled and the liquid drunk. In either case the diuretic action suggested by its popular name 'Piss the Bed' would help to wash out infection and gravel from the kidneys, ureters and bladder and give relief in milder cases of pain and frequency of micturition.

There is one well known treatment for stones, either in the gall bladder or in the urinary tract. I heard this separately from two people in County Galway and it is believed to have come from the monks of Annaghadown. In one case, the treatment gave relief to a lady who suffered from gall stones but was advised that she should not have surgery. The roots of butchers' broom are boiled for eight hours and a pint of whiskey added to a quart of the water. Honey may also be added to sweeten the mixture which is strained and bottled. The patient is instructed to drink three glasses daily and is also told that the whiskey was added to preserve the strength of the decoction. As my informant said:

It melts the kidney stone and every stone in your body.

This appears to be derived from official medicine. K'eogh wrote about butchers' broom:

The root is chiefly used. It is Dieuretic, Lithontroptic and nephritic. The decoction of it breaketh the stone, expelleth the gravel and is very good for them that cannot easily make water.

Another herb, the use of which is still remembered, is crane's bill. I found no details about how it should be prepared, but again K'eogh agrees that it is useful in his usual terms:

It is Dieuretic, Lithontroptic and a great Traumatic. Provokes urine (and) expells the gravel and stone.

There was one preparation, juice of juniper berries, used

simply as a diueretic—to some extent it is still used. K'eogh
gives a long list of the wonderful powers of juniper berries,
one of which is to provoke urine. For retention of urine, a
Mayo treatment is to pulp a turnip and drink the juice.

It would seem from the records of the seventeenth and
eighteenth centuries that diseases of the urinary tract were
much more common then than they are now. In his work on
the Mineral Waters of Ireland, John Rutty makes many
references to patients suffering from the gravel and the
stone who appeared to have benefited from drinking the
different spa waters. In all cases, the waters were drunk in
very large quantities and this no doubt increased the flow of
urine through the kidneys. This would tend to wash out
small fragments of gravel which were causing irritation. Probably more important, the large volume of urine would also
wash out areas of infection in the kidneys and ureters and
so help to relieve milder cases of pyelitis. This treatment is
still used when patients complain of pain and frequency of
micturition; they are advised to drink large quantities of
liquids.

One treatment is still widely used—barley water. The
reference to it in K'eogh sums up its uses at present:

> The decoction of it, being exceeding good in all kinds
> of fevers, in the stone, gravel and heat of urine.

It is often prescribed in infections of the urinary tract. It is
prepared by boiling two ounces of pearl barley in one and a
half pints of water and then straining it. The patient is
encouraged to drink it.

There is a form of treatment for the gravel which may be
descended from the mediaeval Irish system of medicine. It is
prepared by boiling the white heads of the ceannbhán beag
(self heal) with miontas caisil (pellitory of the wall) four
handfuls of each in three pints of water. When boiled for
three hours, the liquid is strained and bottled for use. K'eogh,
as usual, tells about the powers of the two herbs. Of pellitory
of the wall he says:

> It is a great pectoral, a powerful Dieuretic, Lithontroptic
> and nephritic. When there is a stoppage of urine let

the Decoction of it be taken inwardly, or a Poultis of it applyed warm to the region of the bladder.

About self heal he says:

It is a very great Restringent good against internal bleeding and pissing of blood.

There are many treatments for stones in the kidneys or in the bladder to be found in Irish medical manuscripts. This one ordered:

to the groin rub the blood of a fox and it breaks the stones.

CHAPTER V

Whooping Cough

THIS disease may cause serious trouble in children under
one year. From the age of two years onwards it is much less
serious and nearly all patients recover. In some African countries whooping cough is still a very grave disease and a hundred years ago it may have been so in Ireland. This would
account for the large number of cures which are still used.

The disease is ideal for treatment with a folk remedy, or
with any remedy. During the acute phase of the disease, the
sufferer, almost always a child, has severe spasms of coughing
during which, in the eyes of his anxious parents, he appears to
be about to die of asphyxia. The spasm may last for a minute
or more and ends with the characteristic whoop. When the
attack is over the child quickly recovers and seems perfectly
well until another attack occurs. To add to the distress of the
parents—the patient is usually less distressed—the child is
likely to vomit during the attack. The attacks may persist for
some weeks, or even months, and gradually become fewer
until they finally cease, leaving the child in the great majority
of cases none the worse. Sometimes the attacks persist as a
habit.

In such a long drawn out illness, with anxious parents
wondering if their child is going to die in one of the attacks,
many remedies have been used for whooping cough and each
one has its group of enthusiastic believers. After all, official
medicine has used its own share of cures for the condition
and only a few years ago it was advised that the patient be
taken up to ten thousand feet in an airplane with an unpres-
surised cabin. I would have been delighted to welcome this as

a folk cure and record it if I had not read it in a medical
text book.

There is a famous cure for whooping cough used in the area
around the borders of Cavan and Meath. In this case the vault
of a skull reputed to be that of a bishop is kept for the cure. I
have been told that about the year 1830, when an old church
in the neighbourhood was being pulled down, three skulls
were found under the altar and were thought to have been
the skulls of bishops. Two of the skulls have disappeared, but
children suffering from whooping cough are brought from
thirty miles around to drink water from the remaining one.
I have been told that the skull has been taken to England to
treat a case of whooping cough and everyone says that no
child who drank from it ever died of whooping cough.
Certainly people have great faith in this cure, and I was
told of a doctor, noted for his disapproval of folk remedies,
whose daughter unknown to her father was taken to drink
from the skull.

The story about the bishop's skull may have originated in
the seventeenth century for about 1642 an Italian visitor reported to Rome that the relics of Cornelius Devanny, a
martyred Franciscan bishop, were preserved and venerated in
the same neighbourhood.

There are a number of cures which involve husbands and
wives with the same surname. In one of these cures the husband and wife give the first and the last piece of their break-
fasts to the messenger, who takes it to the patient. This cure
was popular in County Leitrim—my parents, who had the
cure, were often asked for it. In County Cavan it is necessary
to visit three such married couples. This is not so difficult in
Cavan, there are comparatively few surnames there. In parts
of Counties Tipperary and Wicklow, the cure is with the
children of parents with the same surname and any piece of
food which the child gives constitutes the cure. Another
County Leitrim cure was begun by giving a meal to a ferret.
Any part of the meal which the ferret did not eat was taken
and given to the patient.

These cures may be very old forms of magic. The personal
factor is of the greatest importance in magical medicine. The
food given by the different people is the vehicle of the magic

and is comparable to the use of breath or fasting spit. There are many other examples of this type of personal magic used in the treatment of whooping cough.

One such method is used in County Clare and I have also heard of it from County Longford. The person seeking the cure, an over-anxious parent perhaps, went out to find a man riding a white horse. When he found such a man the person seeking the cure said to him:

> A fhir an chapaill bháin, cad é an leigheas ar an pioc seo? (Man of the white horse, what is the cure of this disease?)

Whatever he told you to do, you did it, and that constituted the cure. This is another example of personal magic, but one might speculate about why the man riding the white horse became part of the cure. In their book on their tour of Ireland, the Halls remarked that in County Leitrim the doctor always rode a white horse. I failed to find any folk tradition of this custom and it cannot have been known during the twentieth century. It might possibly be a survival from the practice of medicine in mediaeval Ireland when the doctor might have ridden a white horse, but I have not been able to find any contemporary reference to back up this suggestion.

There are many other forms of treatment. Another method, also used in County Leitrim, is to put the winkers of a donkey on the patient, who is then led three times around a pig sty. When this has been completed, those present kneel at the door of the sty and say a few prayers. The origin of this may have been an effort to transfer the disease to the pig, but I have not been able to learn of any words which were said which might suggest this. This method is also used in County Cavan and I have heard of a very intelligent doctor there whose pig sty is conveniently situated and is often used for performing the cure.

What is probably another example of the transference of disease, and a very primitive one, is to have the patient crawl under the belly of an ass foal which has not yet been ridden. Clearly this can be compared to treatments in English folk medicine. Some of these recommend passing the child through a hole in a stone or through a split tree or even through a hole in the ground. All these are examples of an effort to pass the disease on to something else.

Another cure for whooping cough is of interest. To carry it out it is necessary that a piece of red flannel be put on the chest of the patient and, to get the full benefit from this treatment, the red flannel should be put on by the Godfather of the patient. As in so many of these cures, one might speculate about the origin of this one. Why was the child's Godfather involved? And what was the significance of the red flannel? Was it an effort to cast out the devil which was causing the disease?

From west Cork I heard of a cure which consisted of boiling the droppings of sheep in milk and giving the mixture to the patient. The droppings of sheep are recommended by K'eogh as a treatment for many diseases, but not for whooping cough. From west Mayo I have heard that the milk of a donkey is used to treat whooping cough. Again, K'eogh recommends the urine of the donkey for many diseases, but not for whooping cough.

I have only heard of one cough mixture which was used for this disease. This was a mixture of equal parts of white of egg and of honey and it would probably soothe the cough and be of some benefit.

In Dublin there was a cure which must have been used on hundreds of thousands of Dublin children: nearly every Dublin person from whom I enquired knew all about it and many of them had been treated with it. The child was taken to some place where tar was being used and kept there sniffing the hot tar. The usual place was where some convenient road was being tarred, but if this was not possible, the child might be taken to any factory where tar was being used and made to smell it. An alternative Dublin method was to take the child down to the gasometer on the south side of the Liffey, but this was not thought to be as effective as a few hours sniffing the tar. Usually one treatment at the tar was not enough and treatment had to be continued for a number of days.

These wonderful forms of treatment, many of them going back for thousands of years, will soon be forgotten with the control of whooping cough.

CHAPTER VI

Jaundice

JAUNDICE is a very dramatic symptom and one which can be recognised by everyone. The possible causes are many, but by far the most common is infectious hepatitis. At the onset of this disease the patient complains of loss of appetite, abdominal discomfort and depression. These are rather ordinary complaints and little notice might be taken of them by the patient's family, but when after a few days the patient is seen to have turned yellow, then it is time to get some help. Jaundice may be caused by a gall stone which is stopping the flow of bile from the liver to the gut, but this is usually associated with very severe colic pain. In very rare cases the flow of bile may be blocked by a growth, but in this case the jaundice will be much deeper—the black jaundice—as distinct from the yellow jaundice. The significance of this is well recognised by the people who treat jaundice and they say wisely that the black jaundice is not curable. In some cases of infectious hepatitis, the jaundice is much darker than usual and in such a case the medical attendant, qualified or otherwise, may be given the credit for curing the black jaundice. If he is wise, the attendant will be duly modest, otherwise he may find himself expected to cure a case of cancer of the head of the pancreas.

With the dramatic symptom, a sick patient and a very good outlook, the disease is an ideal one for a folk curer or for that matter for any medical attendant. The essential thing is that the attendant should wait for the disease to take its course and, while appearing to be busily engaged in the treatment, do 'nothing in particular but do it very well'.

Masterly inactivity is often the mark of a skilful doctor and in no diseased condition is this more necessary than in the case of a jaundiced patient. For this reason there are many treatments for jaundice, none of which can in any way influence the course of the disease and most of which take about fourteen days to complete.

As in the folk medicine of other countries, yellow plants are prescribed for jaundice in Irish folk medicine. The most usual of these is charlock. This is a bright yellow flower often seen growing in corn. The flowers are boiled and strained and the water drunk. Buttercups are similarly used and once I heard of the use of saffron and the flowers of the yellow iris. Clearly the reason for the use of these plants is their colour. The cure of jaundice by means of yellow things occurs in ancient Indian writings of about three thousand years ago and is also found in an Anglo-Saxon Herbal.

K'eogh recommends both saffron and bastard saffron for jaundice and also the different marigolds, but not charlock. He says:

> A decoction of it (corn marygold) in wine drank, cureth the jaundice. The seed hath the same virtue.

About bastard saffron he said:

> The flowers open obstructions of the liver and are very profitable against the jaundice.

The use of saffron is also advised by Marryat. Turner gives many long prescriptions for the treatment of jaundice and includes saffron in some of them.

In Swedish folklore, a yellowhammer roasted is believed to cure jaundice. K'eogh has this to say about the power of the yellowhammer to cure jaundice:

> Littleton and Cole in their dictionaries tell us that if this bird be looked upon by anyone who has the yellow jaundice, the person is cured but the bird dies.

This legend is also mentioned by Pliny in his Natural History.

I have known of a brother and sister who contracted jaundice at the same time. They were both treated with a preparation of Jew's Ear leaves which were boiled in milk. The girl finished the treatment which took fourteen days and recovered completely, while the boy, who did not complete it, is now the sallow one in a very fair-skinned family.

The treatment of jaundice with boiled worms is still practised and if it is carried out by the seventh son of a seventh son it is especially efficacious. Earthworms are also recommended for jaundice by Turner, and K'eogh says that dried and powdered earthworms cure the jaundice. In his article on the medicinal wonders of earthworms prepared in different ways K'eogh says that they cure almost every disease known and he cannot possibly have believed what he wrote. If a quarter of the things he said were true, there would be no diseases left uncured in Ireland.

Another method, still more disgusting, is the use of powdered lice to treat jaundice. I do not know if this is still used —probably not—but it was used in County Leitrim up to forty years ago. It has a long history of use by official medicine. K'eogh wrote:

> Lice are swallowed alive in an egg by the meaner sort of people to cure jaundice.

About the use of hog lice he wrote:
> The powder of them taken, or swallowed down alive from number three to twelve, for several mornings fasting wonderfully cures the jaundice.

Some more cures may be mentioned. One of these is goose dung boiled in milk. Here again K'eogh may be the source. He wrote:

> The dung (of the goose) is a specific against the jaundice.

Still another ordered that milk mixed with an equal quantity of the patient's urine should be drunk every day for fourteen days. There is another plant also used—the sundew —which grows in bogs. The red leaves are boiled in milk and the decoction drunk daily for at least ten days.

It is clear from the recital of these 'cures' for jaundice— and many more could be given—that the healers served a useful purpose in treating it. They provided what was most necessary—reassurance; and if the forms of treatment often seem disgusting to us, it must be remembered that they were all derived from official medicine. The fact that none of the treatments had any influence on the course of the disease could not be expected to occur to the patient or to his friends. After all, it seems perfectly logical; the patient was ill, the patient was treated, the patient got better. It was probable that the patient was told he was getting such things as goat's dung or earthworms; this would further assure him that he was getting special treatment, and if it were kept up for fourteen days the jaundice would be fading, and the patient well on the way to recovery.

Even if the forms of treatment had no influence on the jaundice, they were much better than the treatment provided by official medicine, which must often have made the patient worse. At the start, the first form of treatment was an emetic. Even Marryat, who was a sensible man, advised this. The emetic was followed by bleeding and very drastic purging, all of which must have added greatly to the patient's discomfort as well as making him worse. The reason behind these heroic forms of treatment was the belief that jaundice was due to some obstruction, somewhere, and the vomiting, bleeding and purging were designed to remove all obstructions wherever they were. After this assault, treatment with worms or lice would be pleasant and could not possibly do any harm. Modern medicine has advanced perhaps a little beyond the folk curer. We now try to make the patient comfortable and are able to reassure him, but in the eyes of the patient our reassurance is hardly more effective than treatment for a fortnight or so with saffron or goose dung.

CHAPTER VII

Headache

HEADACHE is a rather vague word. In the great majority of cases no physical cause can be found for it, and one accepts the word of the patient if he says he has a headache. The attacks vary greatly in severity. It may be no more than a mild annoyance, easily relieved by five grains of aspirin, or a severe attack of migraine, when the pain is so severe that the patient is clearly unable to do his ordinary work and must lie down in the dark. In such severe cases, the patient may see zig-zag patterns of lights and may also vomit or even suffer temporary blindness. Also the pain may be confined to one side of the head. In many of the milder cases the attack may be provoked by a state of anxiety and in fact the word 'headache' may be used as an excuse for almost anything.

In these cases, where the cause is so often functional, many forms of charms and incantations may be used to relieve it —psychotherapy may be used under many disguises. There is a famous incantation to relieve a headache which can be found in a number of manuscripts and seems to be Christian in origin. In this case, the words of the incantation are in Latin and the instructions are given in Irish. It reads:

> Caput Christi, oculus Isaie, frons nassium Noe, Labia lingua Salamonis, Collum Temathei, Mens Benjamen, pectus Pauli, junctus Johannis, fides Abrache, Sanctus, Sanctus, Sanctus, Dominus Deus Sabaoth.

> This is sung every day about thy head against headache. After singing it, thou puttest thy spittle in thy palm and thou puttest it round thy temples and on thy occiput and

thereat thou sayest thy Pater Noster, thrice, and thou
puttest a cross of thy spittle on the crown of thy head
and then thou makest this sign U on thy head.

The Latin text of this charm may also be found in an
English manuscript, Harley 2965, in the British Museum
Library, which was written in the eighth century, so it is
about contemporary with the Irish text. The differences
between the texts are few. I cannot explain the U-shaped
sign which was made on the head, but there is no doubt
that, if the patient were to repeat the words daily and carry
out the prescribed ritual, he would probably benefit psycho-
logically.

There is another ritual for the relief of headache which is
probably still used in many parts of Ireland. I have heard of
its being used in Counties Mayo, Galway and Leitrim. When
the patient consulted the man who made the cure, he first carefully examined the patient's head to learn if the sutures of
the skull were open or not. If they were found to be open, he
then measured the circumference of the head. When all these
preliminaries had been duly completed, he got to work and
by pressing on different points of the head he was able to
press the bones of the sutures together. The pressure was
sufficient to cause some pain to the patient. When this pressing had been continued for some time the healer again
measured the head and in a favourable case found that the
sutures had now been closed. In most cases it was necessary
to carry out the ritual on a number of successive days.

This is a brilliant piece of psychotherapy. The healer will
be sufficiently intelligent and experienced to see if the headaches are mainly functional, so in such a case he is able to
give a good prognosis; on the other hand, he may find that
the sutures are not open, or only slightly open, and then the
prognosis would not be so good. Certainly, if the headaches
are functional in origin, the ritual of measuring and squeezing and the repetition will probably be of great benefit to
the patient. Carried out by a healer who understood people
and sympathised with them, this treatment would surely be
as helpful as the best modern psychotherapy.

There are some other forms of treatment for headache

which could be called routine methods; there is nothing dramatic about them. Strong brown paper soaked in vinegar may be applied to the site of the pain. This would probably be quite refreshing. The paper might also be soaked in whiskey. If one of these treatments is continued for some time—it may be necessary to continue for months—the headaches may be greatly improved.

More energetic measures are sometimes necessary. I have heard a story about one patient who had his head shaved and a mustard blister applied. It is likely that, having submitted to such treatment once, the patient might decide to say nothing further about headaches for fear of having the treatment repeated. Burgundy pitch may also be used as a counter-irritant. I was assured that the pains were relieved by the shaving and blistering. The most usual folk remedy was to rub the forehead and temples with the leaves of crowfoot. These leaves are strong counter-irritants and could cause severe blistering. The person performing the cure was probably able to judge the correct amount of rubbing best suited to each case. It is likely that recurring headaches have been relieved by visiting holy wells, drinking the water, doing the prescribed station and praying to the saint. Saint Fechin's well at Fore, County Westmeath, is famous and many cases of chronic headache have been relieved there.

The shaving of the head and blistering has a long history. Marryat advised a blister over the whole head or a plaster of Burgundy pitch applied to the temples.

In a case record taken from a book by a distinguished seventeenth century Irish doctor, Edmund O'Meara, the shaving and blistering for headache is described. I have taken the liberty of translating the Latin text. It begins:

Headache and running of the eyes cured by
Blistering, and an outbreak of
Small Pox.

A very excellent lady, Miss Mary More, a member of the family of the illustrious Thomas More, formerly Lord Chancellor of England, consulted me at Bath. She had suffered for many years from dimness of vision, with running eyes and headache. When different remedies had been tried and she had bathed the eyes and used the baths in vain, I applied a strong blister to her shaven head from the front to the back. This caused great vesicles to form. The headache disappeared (temporarily) and was not very severe when it recurred, and the dimness of vision completely disappeared. Although a great quantity of serous humour was removed in two days by the blister, the running of the eyes remained and I could hope to cure this by means of some of the usual remedies. When the flow increased to a waterfall, I advised her that she might expect the return of him who caused it at a proper and suitable time. Not many days afterwards she developed small pox with the eruption mainly on the head, and when the eruption cleared, the cause of the running eyes was also removed as I think very likely by the small pox so that ever since she has been happily free from both diseases.

Closing the sutures of the skull or repeating an incantation are pleasant forms of treatment compared with that given to Miss More by her distinguished physician.

CHAPTER VIII

The Mouth and Throat

APHTHOUS ULCERS

These are small ulcers which occur on the mucous membrane which covers the inside of the mouth. They are often painful and a considerable source of annoyance to the patient. The treatment used in County Leitrim was to swab them with a mixture of honey and borax. This would give some relief. They may also be swabbed with vinegar.

THRUSH

This is an infection of the lining of the mouth and tongue with a yeast-like fungus called monilia. It may not have been a very common infection in rural Ireland up to thirty years ago—babies were not bottle fed or treated with antibiotics, the two great causes of the condition. The cases which occurred were associated with poor general care of the baby and when the standard of care improved the infection was likely to clear up. It appears as white patches and on discovering it the parents are greatly disturbed and will immediately look for help.

A very simple treatment may be given by a man who never saw his own father; he simply breathes over the patient's mouth. In some cases the healer must be a seventh son, but the treatment is the same and, in cases when these healers are not easily available, the breathing may be done by a fasting gander. In addition to the breathing, it is advised that the white patches be cleaned off the inside of the mouth. This would go a great way towards clearing up the condition.

The curing of a disease by breathing on the sufferer is very old in medicine. Tertullian wrote that heathen spirits feared the touch and the breath of man. In pagan Rome it was believed that evil spirits were the cause of disease and could be driven out by breathing on the sick person. Perhaps the reason why this form of treatment continued in use here was because Our Lord breathed on His apostles when leaving His power to them. I am unable to suggest any reason why the breath of a fasting gander was credited with the power to cure thrush.

MUMPS

This disease presents itself dramatically with a swelling on each cheek just in front of and below the ear. When the parents see the swelling, they will immediately seek treatment, and, as the prognosis of this disease in young children is very good, there will be no difficulty in finding it. Even if it does not do much good for the patient, it will help the parents.

Some people would advise that the winkers of an ass be put on the patient and that he be led to a convenient river where he must drink the water. It is important that the water be drunk directly from the river, not from any drinking vessel. Another version says that the patient, wearing the winkers, must be led across a south flowing stream, or he may be led three times around a pig-sty (cró muice). Those making the cure may then kneel at the door of the sty and say some prayers. This method is also used for the treatment of whooping cough.

A more dramatic form of treatment has been used in County Meath. I have heard of a lady who came to visit a child who was suffering from mumps. When she had seen the child, she went out to the pig-sty and was overheard saying to the pig:

> A mhuic, a mhuic, chugat an leicneach seo.
> (Pig, pig, here, take the mumps.)

This lady did not know the meaning of her words or that she was speaking Irish. A slightly different method is that the person performing the cure stands with her back against the door jamb and, standing as tall as possible, says the same words—this is the method used in County Westmeath.

These cures are examples of transference. Clearly, the old lady was transferring the disease to the pig. Leading the patient to the flowing water and having him drink it may be an effort to transfer the disease to the water. The use of running water to carry away evil is very old and is found in the Saxon leechbooks. Probably the river flowing to the south makes the cure still more powerful. The leading around the pig-sty may also be an effort to transfer the disease to the pig. 'Cró' also means an enclosure for domestic animals, so originally the ritual might have been to lead the patient around this enclosure.

SORE THROAT

Nearly everyone has at some time or other suffered from an acute infection of the tonsils. The infection is both painful and sickening and the patient feels very miserable. In such cases, one form of treatment is to fill a worsted stocking with hot salt and put this as a collar around the painful area. When skilfully prepared and applied, this will give some relief. Another method is to fill the stocking with hot potatoes. Some minor variations of these methods of applying a counter-irritant are found. It may be necessary to use the stocking that the patient has been wearing. In other diseases a silk or nylon stocking, in which the caterpillar of the butterfly (Hairy Molly) has been wrapped may also be used.

Another method is to use Saint Brigid's Cotton. In this case a piece of cotton cloth which had been left outside the door of the house on the night before the first of February is used. This is the Feast of Saint Brigid and the story is that the saint as she passed by blessed the cloth. The cloth is tied around the painful throat.

CHRONIC SORE THROAT

Chronic sore throats are also common, but in these cases there is a different form of treatment. When the healer examines the throat he may find that the small tongue (the uvula) has fallen down and it is necessary to put it back in its proper place. It is true that the uvula may become infected and in such a case it will appear longer than usual due to the swelling. People still believe that if the uvula were ever to touch the back of the tongue the patient would die.

In many of these cases there is a large emotional element and therefore it may be possible to touch the uvula, the back of the tongue, and the throat, without causing any discomfort to the patient. The person making the cure can press on the uvula and after some such manoeuvring is able to assure the patient that it has been replaced and he is now out of danger. In some cases this manoeuvring is not possible and another method must be tried. The curer now examines the crown of the patient's head in search of a certain hair which he alone knows where to find and who is able to recognise it when he has found it. It is believed that this special hair is attached to the uvula and the curer is able to replace it by pulling on the hair.

The swelling and lengthening of the uvula was described by Celsus and by the tenth century it had been taken into Saxon medicine. It may be presumed to have been part of old Irish medicine but I have not seen any very early references to it. In almost every case it is a harmless condition and requires no treatment. Unfortunately, it could become the centre of a difficult neurosis.

There are some other treatments which might help. Gargling with salt and water is popular and I met one case in which a solution of perchloride of iron was used to gargle. This has been taken directly from official medicine. A solution of two ounces of Friar's Balsam in a pint of water is boiled in a steam kettle and the steam inhaled.

Blocked sinuses were treated by chewing bees' wax. I do not know what effect, if any, this might have, but it was the recognised method in County Cavan. Sneezing was prevented or cured by holding a coal from a turf fire under the nose of the sufferer who inhaled the smoke. Once I saw this being done and the sneezing stopped.

CHAPTER IX

The Eyes

THE earliest Irish reference to eye disease and its treatment will be found in the Life of Saint Columba by Adamnan. A certain Colga, son of Cellach, asked the saint for and was given a piece of rock salt which Columba had blessed. This was to be used by his sister and by his nurse who were suffering from severe inflammation of the eyes.

An ancient charm for the treatment of sore eyes can be found written on a margin of the Stowe Missal. It is in old Irish and the part of it which can be read has been translated:

> I honour bishop Ibar who heals . . . may the blessing of God and of Christ's . . . heal thine eye . .   whole of thine eye. Haec cum dixisset in terram et fecit etc. (John IX. 7.)

In this case the charm is based on the miracle of Our Lord described in Chapter IX of Saint John's Gospel when He healed a blind man by putting clay mixed with spittle on his eyes.

In the records of the eighteenth and nineteenth centuries, eye diseases appear to have been common in Ireland. Many people were blinded by small pox, but the most important cause of eye diseases may have been the smoke which must have been a grave nuisance in the houses of poor people, when efficient chimneys were rare and sometimes there was no chimney at all.

One of the most popular forms of treatment for sore eyes was to bathe them in the water of certain holy wells. Saint

Patrick's Well on the side of Slieve an Iarrain in County
Leitrim was well known. Saint Catherine's Well near Killy-
begs, and another well near Lacken in County Wicklow
also cure sore eyes. Still others are Saint Brigid's Well near
Mulhuddart in County Dublin and Saint Brigid's Well near
Ballyheigue in County Kerry. Perhaps the most famous of
the holy wells is in the townland of Tully near Ballygar in
County Galway. The story goes that early in the nineteenth
century a man named Kelly living in the neighbourhood had
a daughter twenty-one years old who had been born blind.
He dreamed that his daughter should go to the well and
bathe her eyes in the water. She did this and her sight was
restored. Ever since, people have been visiting the well, the
water of which still continues to cure sore eyes.

STY

There are a large number of treatments for stys, most of
which are continued while the infection runs its natural
course and then clears up. A very simple one is probably part
of a children's game. If someone says to the patient: 'There
is a sty on your eye', the sufferer may cure it by saying: 'You
lie'. Another method is to make the Sign of the Cross over
the sty with the marriage ring of the patient's mother. It was
necessary to repeat this daily for nine days. As has been
noticed, marriage rings are used in many folk cures. Another
old form of treatment widely used in folk medicine is to rub
the infected area with fasting spit and, as in the other uses
of fasting spit, the treatment must be repeated daily for the
usual nine days.

A treatment which is practiced in many parts of Ireland
is the use of a twig of a gooseberry bush with nine thorns. All
the other thorns are broken off the twig until only nine
remain and care is taken to see that each thorn points in
the direction opposite to the thorn next to it. Each thorn in
turn is pointed at the sty and an Our Father, a Hail Mary
and a Gloria are said each time. The ritual is repeated daily
for nine days to complete the cure.

The use of the number nine is part of the ancient leech
lore of the Irish and is often found in modern folk medicine.
In an ancient law tract dealing with wounds it is laid down

that the patient must be examined by a doctor on the ninth day after an injury. In another medico-legal tract the nine doors of the soul are mentioned and in an eighth century poem Our Lord is praised because He healed people without waiting for nine days as the doctors did. There are also many references to nines in the Saxon Leechbooks. In any case, the sty would be well on the way to being healed at the end of nine days, if treated by fasting spit or with nine gooseberry thorns, or by any other method.

Two other forms of treatment may be of interest. The sty may be bathed with the milky juice of the dandelion. It may also be bathed with cold tea.

SORE EYES

The treatments for the sty may be used for sore eyes in general. There are also other treatments for sore eyes. The eyes may be bathed with the juice of a plant called tourpin. This is the house leek (semper vivum tectorum), which is sometimes seen growing on the wall of a house which it is believed to protect against fire.

In the graveyard of the ruined church of Kiltoghert in County Leitrim, a certain Franciscan friar, Father John MacKeon, is buried. This man had been Guardian of the Franciscan Friary of Jamestown and before his death he is reputed to have said that after his death people would take the clay from his grave to cure sore eyes. When I visited the grave about twenty years ago, it was quite evident that clay had been taken in considerable quantities from it. I learned that the clay is prepared by the same method as Our Lord used when he mixed clay with spittle and used it to restore sight to a blind man.

MOTES

In the area of the Sligo/Mayo border there is a charm used to take a mote out of an eye. It was not necessary that the lady who made the cure should be present and examine the eye. When the accident occurred, a messenger was sent to the curer to ask her to treat the condition. When she had been told of the case, she took a saucer of water and prayed over it for some time. When the prayers were ended she looked in the water and if the mote had come out of the eye she saw it in the water. If she could not see the mote it might mean that the mote was still in the eye or that it had come out before the messenger arrived.

This charm may be a version of one recorded in the Saxon Leechbooks for 'worms in the eyes'. The patient must sit with a saucer of water on each side of him and by jerking his head from side to side the worms will fall into the water.

There are more modern methods of getting out motes. I saw a lady expertly turn up an upper eyelid and flick off the mote with a piece of cotton wool. I have heard of, but have not seen, a mote being licked out. This might possibly work if something like a small piece of grit got stuck in the cornea.

I have heard of a method of preventing blindness which may be very old. The patient gets a rush and makes a small loop with it. The loop is filled with a film of spittle and if the patient looks through the film he will never go blind.

I must confess I cannot suggest any reason for the belief that having a pea at the back of the neck while the patient is drawing water is good for weak eyes. I have also heard people say that children should not be allowed to wear glasses; if their eyes need a correction they will grow out of it if they do not wear the glasses. Another method of preserving the sight is to bathe the eyes in the dew. And finally, a black eye may be treated by putting a piece of raw sheep's liver over the bruise and keeping it there with a bandage.

CHAPTER X

The Worm

In Anglo-Saxon primitive medical magic there are many references to diseases which were believed to have been caused by worms. Singer has written that 'the doctrine of the worm' is one of the four elements which distinguish native Teutonic medicine and magic. The others are the doctrine of specific venoms, the doctrine of the nines and the doctrine of the elf-shot. There is evidence to show that the doctrine of the nines and the doctrine of the elf-shot were also part of primitive Celtic magic medicine, and it would seem that the ancient Irish believed that worms caused certain diseases.

In Anglo-Saxon, the word 'wyrm' may mean a worm, an insect, a snake or a dragon. 'Flaesc-wyrm' is a flesh worm or maggot. In Irish, an ordinary word for a worm is 'piast' and the word also means a maggot, an intestinal worm or an insect, especially a stinging insect. Other words in Irish are 'míl-cheartán' which means a flesh worm, i.e. a worm which infects the flesh. Dineen quotes the expression:

Ta mílcheárda i mbonna mo chos
(there are flesh worms in the soles of my feet).

'Cnuimh' also means a worm or a maggot.

I have heard one example of the belief in worms as a cause of disease in modern Irish folk medicine. In County Kerry boils may be treated with a poultice made of the boiled root of comfrey. When I asked why this was done, I was surprised to learn that the poultice was used to drive the worms out of the boil. They are unable to tolerate the smell of the poultice and therefore they run away.

In a charm written in old Irish against toothache, the sufferer asked for protection against worms and pangs. The same idea is conveyed in modern Irish by the reference to

an phiast atá im' fhiacail (the worm in my tooth).

In a sixteenth century treatise, on diseases of horses, in the Irish language there is one reference to worms as a cause of disease:

We come now to sibus, which consists of worms which grow from the jaw upwards and when it goes (or they go) into the ear, the horse goes mad and dies, and the right treatment is to burn it with this iron.

The word translated 'worms' is 'cruma' (modern Irish, 'cnuimhe'). I do not know exactly what disease is meant by the word 'sibus', but it may be some acute infection of the jaw and certainly, if the infection spreads to the ear, a brain abscess is quite likely to occur and the horse would certainly go mad and die.

In one of the Saxon Leechbooks, the Lacnunga, there is a charm called 'the worm charm', which is to be recited

in case a man or a beast drink a wyrm.

The first three words of the charm are, surprisingly, in Irish and read:

Gonomil, orgomil, marbumil.

In modern Irish this probably would be:

Goin an míol, airg an míol, marbhaigh an míol
(Wound the worm, harass the worm, kill the worm).

One might speculate about how this charm became part of Anglo-Saxon magic. Perhaps some of the Irish monks had a reputation as a medicine man, and in any case it is an example of the survival of a forgotten language.

In a primitive society, worms might seem a more obvious cause of disease than would be the case today. Anyone could see that maggots and flies caused serious disease in sheep and in cattle. Maggots could be found in wounds of animals and cannot have been very rare in human wounds.

In Irish folk medicine, a seventh son is credited with the power to heal many diseases; as proof of his power, it is said that he kills worms by touching them. I well remember when, as a young boy, I went digging for worms I was told that it was unwise to have a seventh son help to pick the worms because if he touched them they would all die. An imaginative older companion assured me that his worms had been killed in that way, and even if one only half believed the story there was no sense in taking any chance.

In a general way there was a fear of the harm which worms might cause. In County Leitrim I was often warned about a legendary creature called a man-creeper which lived in water and might get into the body through the sole of the foot, or in through the mouth if one drank bad water. Here there may have been confusion with the leech, because it was said that the man-creeper might suck blood. Other dangerous creatures were the earwig, which might get into the brain through the ears, and the conach worm, which was reputed to cause disease in cattle.

These few references to worms as a cause of disease show that this belief was held by the Irish as well as by the Teutonic tribes.

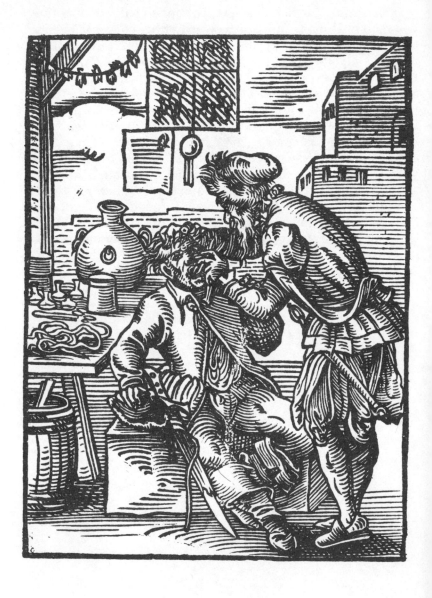

Part 2

External Ailments

CHAPTER I

Skin Diseases

'When I was a student there were only two skin diseases,
The one you cured with sulphur and the one you didn't.'

I REMEMBER this quotation from a book called 'Horse and
Buggy Doctor' by Albert Hertzler, who practiced in Kansas
around 1880. It may have been an over-simplification of the
case, but he also wrote that itch was the only disease which
doctors could cure when he was a boy. In any case, people
generally are much more worried about a mild skin rash,
which the patient can see, than about a more serious disease
which he cannot see. The fact that often skin diseases are
on the face or the hands so that everybody else can see them
is more important still. For these reasons it will be understood why there are so many forms of treatment for this
group of diseases and so many advertised treatments for
pimples, acne, blackheads, etc., which are such a source of
anxiety to adolescents.

NETTLE STINGS

As children are usually the ones who get stung by nettles,
the treatment is suitably designed for them. When the child
gets stung, it is necessary to find a fresh dock leaf. These can
almost always be found around houses where nettles are also
likely to be found. The pain of the sting only lasts for a few
minutes, so that by the time a dock leaf is found the pain
will have begun to get less. In order to increase the effect, it
is necessary that the sufferer also say some suitable words
and keep repeating them while rubbing with the leaf. A few
examples will illustrate the routine:

1) Dock, Dock, you cure me and I'll cure you.
2) Dockin, Dockin, sting nettle.
3) Dockin, Dockin in and out
Take the sting of the nettle out.

and here is a version in Irish:

4) Neanntóg a thoit mé,
Biolar sraide leighis mé
(a nettle burned me, dock cure me).

BEE STINGS

A sting by a bee or a wasp is much more painful than a nettle sting and usually an effort is made to get the sting out if it can be seen. When this is done, the painful area may be rubbed with the raw surface of an onion. The more usual treatment, which is used in most parts of Ireland, is to rub the painful area with a blue bag. I have been told that the blue is used more now for treating bee stings than for its original use—blueing clothes.

CHILBLAINS

Medical attendants sometimes regard chilblains as of little importance, an opinion shared by people who have not suffered from them. To those who suffer from chilblains they are of great importance and indeed, if the skin breaks, they can prevent the patient from working. Schoolboys have a very simple treatment for chilblains: they micturate on them and are certain that this relieves the pain and itching. If this is not possible, the painful areas may be bathed in fresh urine. A slightly more orthodox method is to bathe the hands or feet in forge water. This is the water kept in a stone trough in a forge and is used by the smith to cool hot iron. The chilblains may also be painted with cod liver oil or dressed with a piece of lint soaked in the cod liver oil. I do not know if it is still prescribed, but about forty years ago cod liver oil taken orally was an official treatment for chilblains.

ITCH

The use of sulphur for the treatment of itch is probably the oldest form of treatment still in use. It is only in

the past few years, after more than two thousand years of
success, that official medicine has found more efficient forms
of treatment. The itch can cause great difficulties in com-
munities like armies and logging camp gangs and in army
hospitals there was usually a special itch ward. The standard
treatment is an ointment made of sulphur and hog's lard.
This is recommended by Turner, who says that poor people
drink flowers of sulphur in milk:

> anointing outwardly at the same time with the flowers
> of brimestone mixed up with butter or Hog's lard.

The rich were, of course, purged, bled and sweated, and
probably as an incidental got a box of sulphur ointment
which would cure the disease. Everybody agreed that sulphur
cured itch but a rich patient might be given it by mouth. I
remember well being rubbed with sulphur ointment but
I was also given a preparation of sulphur and treacle by
mouth. The itch mite was shown at a meeting of the Dublin
Philosophical Society about the year 1685 by Thomas
Molyneux, but in 1764 'The New Practice of Physic' by
Thomas Marryat said:

> The cause is an infectious miasma sui generis. The old
> notion of animalcules is justly exploded.

CORNS

An ivy leaf tied around a soft corn is said to cure it—if
the treatment can be continued for long enough. A more
elaborate treatment is to soak the feet in a strong solution
of washing soda. This is repeated daily for several days until
the pain of the corn is relieved. If these methods are not
successful, a handful of ivy leaves should be put to steep in
a pint of vinegar in a tightly corked bottle for forty-eight
hours. The liquid is then poured off and still kept tightly
corked. When required, it is applied carefully to each corn,
taking care to see that the preparation does not get on the
skin—it is very painful, K'eogh has this to say about the
therapeutic uses of ivy leaves:

> the juice of the leaves cures wounds, ulcers, burns and
> scalds.

The use of vinegar (a 5.4% solution of acetic acid) in the treatment of corns is an efficient method, and, if persisted in, would probably remove the corn completely. It was not a very popular remedy because it was liable to cause considerable pain. The most usual method was to bathe the corn in hot water and pare it with a razor. The corn was then touched with a drop of carbolic acid.

ERYSIPELAS

Saint Anthony's Fire or Wild Fire usually occurs on the face. It is due to a streptococcal infection of the skin and the infected areas are red and raised. The distribution has been compared to a map of the west of Scotland. In acute cases the patient is extremely ill and before penicillin was available there was a possibility that he might die.

As might be expected, there were several forms of treatment available for the condition. In County Leitrim a thick coat of white paint might be put on the face. As the paint dried it might to some extent act as a splint and help to immobilise the part. This could possibly help to stop the spread of the infection to fresh areas of skin. The area might also be treated with a poultice of fresh cow dung. This treatment may be derived from K'eogh who wrote:

> A cataplasm or Poultis made of the fresh dung (of a calf) is proper to be applied to an erysipililas or St. Anthony's fire.

A most notable form of treatment is the use of Keogh's blood. The cure is possessed by a family called Keogh who live near Two Mile House in County Kildare. In making this cure, a male member of the family rubs some of his own blood on the infected area and this quickly cures it. This cure is widely known in Counties Wicklow, Kildare and Carlow and everybody believes in its usefulness. The use of blood as a method of treating disease is very ancient and will be discussed later.

LIP HERPES

This is usually a trivial disease but it can be quite painful. In County Leitrim people say that it is caused by the urine of a mouse. The expression is: 'I see the mouse p - - - d on you.' Usually there is no treatment given in milder cases. In severe cases the name of the sufferer is written with pen and ink around the painful area.

SHINGLES (*Herpes Zoster*)

This is a very painful condition. The patient complains of severe pain, usually in a localised area of some part of the head, face or trunk. On examination, nothing is seen, but in about forty-eight hours large numbers of blisters appear on the painful area.

One very intelligent form of treatment was practiced in County Mayo. The person making the cure applied zinc ointment to the painful area. This was helped out with ten Our Fathers and ten Hail Marys said by the person making the cure along with the patient. The ointment was applied and the prayers repeated daily by the patient and his medical attendant for ten days and it was stressed that in the case of a male patient the curer must be a female, and vice versa. By the end of ten days the pain would have got very much less and the blisters would be reduced to scabs which were beginning to fall off. The people making the cure always insisted that treatment must be started as early as possible. This is wise, because there is a slight danger that the pain may persist for a longer time in some elderly patients. This cure shows an excellent knowledge of the natural history of the disease and of the psychology of the patient.

Another method is used in County Sligo—a very simple one. The person making the cure inspected the blisters and was able to judge the stage which the disease had then reached. He next touched the blisters and gave his prognosis. This was usually that the pain would get worse for a day or so and then begin to get less and gradually disappear completely. The accurate prognosis is the important thing in this case and naturally people are impressed by it.

Shingles may also be treated with the fasting spit of the person making the cure, who rubs it on the blisters. Fasting spit has an important place in the history of medicine and it is used for many conditions. When the spit has been applied, the Sign of the Cross is made over the blisters with a wedding ring. The virtue of the wedding ring, in this and in other such cures, is due to the fact that it has been blessed.

ECZEMA IN CHILDHOOD

This is often a great trouble to the parents and sometimes to the child. One popular method of treatment is to use no soap on the baby: this is the popular Dublin cure and it is often effective. Another method was to consult a seventh son, or better still, the seventh son of a seventh son. Usually the curer explained to the parents that treatment must be prolonged, but if the parents persist the condition will heal without scarring—it always does—but the parents will be greatly relieved to hear it. Some different preparations are used. A mixture of equal parts of honey and thick cream has been advised and used. Honey mixed with thick buttermilk (curds) is also used. Unsalted butter to which the juice of cabbage has been added is another preparation, and there are many more.

Unfortunately, the scratching often causes the eczematous areas to become secondarily infected and this is a more difficult problem. Most of the older preparations which could be used to clear up the secondary infections were irritating and that made the eczema worse. Here is one which looks as if it had been taken from official medicine:

ointment of lead subacetate	$1\frac{1}{2}$ oz.
ointment of tar	2 drams
ointment of mercury nitrate	2 drams
ointment of zinc oxide to	4 ozs.

This was popular in County Longford and certainly would help to clear the secondary infection. In general the less irritation the better, and a mixture of equal parts of zinc ointment and vaseline is probably the best of all the folk preparations for eczema.

There is some evidence that psychotherapy was used to treat the condition. The patient may be told to drink a quart of milk daily. Another such cure is that the patient must only drink goat's milk and I have heard of a patient whose eczema cleared up on the goat's milk. In any case, sooner or later the condition clears up. One case I remember well is that of a perfectly behaved child, who never cried, and always took his feed, but wheezed and suffered from eczema. When he got big enough—at age three years—to attack his parents and his sister, the wheezing stopped and the eczema cleared up.

ECZEMA IN ADULTS

This is a difficult problem. One preparation, which has been used with some success, is an ointment of archangel tar and mutton suet.

A bran poultice is often used to treat dry eczematous patches and other chronic skin diseases. The bran is first treated with boiling water and then made into a soft paste. This was applied daily, usually for a week, and has been found very useful in some cases.

IMPETIGO

Up to thirty years ago many children and adults suffered from staphlococcal infections of the skin which were called, in a general way, impetigo. It might present itself as large crusts on the scalp and face, or elsewhere, and was quite unsightly. There were many forms of treatment but, before anything else, the hair was clipped short and the crusts carefully cleaned off with warm water. One form of treatment from County Cavan is well worth recording. In this case three children of one family had the infection on their feet and legs. They were told to run up and down in their bare feet in the drain which ran from the cow byre and the infection quickly cleared up with a few such treatments. If the infection happened to be on the face or the scalp the contents of the drain was gathered up—a mixture of urine and cow dung—and the areas bathed with it.

A less bucolic form of treatment was a poultice of oat meal and buttermilk. An ointment, popular in County Meath, is used to treat many skin conditions including impetigo. This ointment contains mercury and lard and is probably a folk version of the official mercury ointment. It would be quite effective in clearing up impetigo.

RINGWORM

There are more cures for ringworm than for any other

condition treated by folk medicine. It is likely that there are many conditions included. In practice any skin disease which took something like a ring form and did not clear up quickly was called ringworm. More exactly, it is a condition caused by a fungus infection of the skin. It is caused by a number of related organisms some of which also cause infection in domestic animals, so cross-infection between animals and man is quite common.

One form of treatment is to put Friar's Balsam on the infected areas daily for about a week. When this has been done, the areas are then treated daily with linseed oil. Black ink was also used. This was first applied in a ring around each patch and inside the ring it was applied first in the form of a cross. The entire area was then treated with the ink and all this with a number of prayers brought about the cure. Another form of treatment—this time from County Wexford—was an ointment made of lard, to which the tobacco ashes from a pipe had been added. Another ointment made of unsalted butter and juice of laurel leaves was also used, but, in addition, prayers were recited. The soft pith of the elder tree was gathered and made into a poultice with cream and applied to the ringworm patches.

A friend of mine is liable to become quite indignant when he remembers all the doctors who tried to cure his ringworm. It was finally cleared in a few days by means of a bread poultice.

A mixture of turpentine and bread soda is also used to treat ringworm and, in the best tradition of folk medicine, an ointment made of goose dung and hog lard.

One ointment, clearly derived from official medicine is still used in County Longford. It consists of:

Amoniated mercury ointment	2 drams
Salicyic acid	30 grains
Yellow paraffin wax to	1 ounce

Psychotherapy may also be used in what must often have been a most intractable condition. Some people believe that it is cured by the touch of a seventh son, in other cases it must be touched by the seventh son of a seventh son, and in still others it must be the touch of a seventh daughter, who also makes the Sign of the Cross over it. Straw from the Christmas crib is kept and used to make the Sign of the Cross over the patches. In another treatment the healer just placed his thumb on the infected area for some minutes and in a few days the patch dried up and the crusts fell off. If all these methods have failed, the patient may be taken to a stable and a saddle strapped on his back.

It must be clear that there were many different conditions which were called ringworm in rural Ireland. Some of these responded to good psychotherapy, for it is difficult to account otherwise for the success of so many forms of treatment.

THE ROSE

A few miles from Bailieborough in County Cavan there is a dried-up lake which was called Lough Leighis (the Healing Lake). During the eighteenth century the water and mud of this lake had a great reputation for curing all sorts of skin diseases. Rutty had this to say about it:

> The water of Lough Leighis, however, in the year 1736 was resorted to from all parts of this Kingdom, and even from England, as an infallable remedy in Cuteneous Eruptions and ulcers: and the very mud of it was exported for these purposes: and indeed whatever virtues are deducible from a fat unctious mud the waters of this lough may lay claim to.

Rutty also says that the lake water was first used for curing the mange in horses and dogs.

The bog mud from the bed of the lake is still used to treat what is called the rose (rosacea). It must be collected at midnight and used as a face-pack. If treatment is continued daily for some weeks the condition, which is sometimes an embarrassment to the sufferers, will be significantly improved.

Poultices of bog mud as a treatment for skin diseases are used in many parts of Ireland. The mud of some bogs appears to be more effective than others—the best muds are free from clay and from small sticks and, mixed with water, make a smooth paste. The wet mud is applied as a face-pack and must be kept moist while it is being used.

FLESH BRUSH

When I was a boy, I was shown what was called a flesh brush. It was about the size and shape of a hand, with a strap across the back like the brush used to groom a horse. The bristles were set very closely together and may have been pig bristles. It was used to brush the skin and remove scruf and scales and many people said they felt very much better for a good brushing—'it toned up the entire system'. I have not heard of it for many years but probably there is some modern version still being used.

INGROWING TOE NAILS

This is a common condition and one which can be quite disabling. Years ago I knew a man who was advised by his brother, a doctor, to have the nails of both his great toes removed. Instead, he went to a neighbour who did some efficient chiropody on him and then taught him how to continue with the treatment. Once a week he had to wash his feet and dry them thoroughly. He then cut the toe nails carefully, taking special care with the painful edge. When this had been done, the neighbourhood of the nail was swabbed with methylated spirits and finally the area was painted with strong tincture of iodine. The patient ended his story: 'and that's ten years ago and I never had any trouble with my feet since'.

CHICKEN POX

This is a mild disease which requires little treatment, but sometimes a few small pitted scars are left, which may cause some embarrassment if they are on the face. In order to prevent this pitting, the pocks may be treated with bread soda, which, I was assured, prevents the scarring. Another method of treating the pocks is with an ointment containing the ashes of burnt rushes and gun-powder made up in hog lard. No doubt, the sulphur in the gun-powder would be of some value and also the fine carbon might help.

BEAUTY TREATMENTS

There are, of course, a whole series of beauty treatments which form a part of Irish folk medicine. A simple one is to rub the skin with the raw surface of a cucumber, which was done to remove freckles. Whether it would do that or not is doubtful, but it probably would have a pleasant effect on the skin of the face. A standard method of improving the complexion was to bathe the face with fresh urine. As urine is essentially a solution of salt and water, it could be of some help, and K'eogh has this to say:

> Urine eases the gout the grieved parts being bathed therewith.

A more elegant method of improving the complexion is to use the juice of comfrey root; the root is macerated and the juice pressed out as needed. It has an astringent action and would be quite pleasant on the skin.

Preparations of oat meal were used as beauty treatments in many parts of Ireland. A lotion is prepared by half filling a bottle with meal and filling up the bottle with water. The meal is shaken up regularly by inverting the bottle and the soaking is continued for twenty-four hours, when the water is poured off and used as a skin lotion. This preparation had many names—'sowans', 'white water' and 'bull's milk' are three. As well as a general beauty treatment, the white water was used to treat some minor rashes and its use recalls that of oat meal soap, once a popular toilet soap. In some cases, a poultice of thick buttermilk and oat meal was prepared and used as a face-pack. This treatment would certainly improve such conditions as greasy skin, blackheads and seborrhoeic dermatitis.

THE GREEN PLASTER

A preparation known as 'the green plaster' was widely used in County Mayo to treat many conditions. These include warts, sores, 'bad feet' and skin infections of all sorts. The prescription was:

Three pence worth of Bees wax
    „   „   „   „ White Resin
    „   „   „   „ Hog's Lard
    „   „   „   „ Burgundy Pitch
    „   „   „   „ Verdigris
One glass of sweet oil

The first five ingredients were boiled together and mixed thoroughly. It was then left to set a little and the sweet oil was added and mixed. It must be kept air-tight and used in small quantities.

The values are about those of the year 1890.

STONE BRUISE

Another injury which needed special attention was called in Irish bonn bhualadh, and in English, a stone bruise. This was an injury—usually to the sole of the foot—in people who went barefoot. It was caused by some injury and as the skin on the sole of the foot was very tough it was not broken but the injury caused bleeding under the skin. This appeared as a plum-coloured raised area, hence its Irish name, and was often quite painful. In treatment, care was taken to see that the skin did not break because if it did the wound was certain to become infected. If it was very painful or very large, a dressing soaked in a saturated solution of Glauber's salts was applied.

CHAPTER II

Skin Growths

SKIN growths are classified as benign or malignant. Warts are benign skin growths and it is not very difficult to treat plain or juvenile warts in children or adults. It is more difficult however to treat a large single wart which may occur in either children or adults. If the wart should have a suitable shape, the simplest form of treatment is to tie a horse hair around the narrow base. This, if properly tied, will cut off the blood supply to the wart, causing it to shrivel up and fall off. Turner mentions a man in ancient Rome who treated such warts by sucking them for a time and then at a suitable moment biting them off.

Cauterization is a more drastic method, but, as the wart itself is insensitive to pain, it may be done without any anaesthetic. I once saw this demonstrated by an expert, on himself. He used a piece of steel knitting needle, about half the usual length, with one end stuck on a cork which he used as a handle. The end of the needle was heated in the flame of a candle and he then went to work on the wart which was conveniently situated on the back of his left hand. As far as I can remember, he stroked the crown of the wart gently with the hot needle, but I did not learn what the final result of the treatment was.

A more usual method was to rub these warts with a stick of caustic soda. This was the method used by the men who worked in the Gas Works in Dublin and who were liable to develop what they called 'Pitch Warts' on their hands. Apart from the rubbing with caustic soda, they paid little attention to them and they had no fear that the warts might become cancerous.

It is of interest to find each of these three methods mentioned by Turner in his book on skin diseases (1736). About the first method he says:

> If the wart be of the pensile kind and seated safely I prefer the ligature made of an Horse-hair or a strong waxed Thread or Silk.

When this has been done he continued:

> After which if necessary the root may be just singed with a red hot probe or knitting-needle.

I do not know if caustic soda was used in medicine in the early years of the eighteenth century, but oil of vitriol (sulphuric acid) could be used and lunar caustic (silver nitrate) was prepared in the form of a stick and used in the same way as caustic soda.

CANCER OF THE SKIN

The treatment of skin cancer is one of the specialities of folk medicine and one where for long the folk curer enjoyed considerable success. Usually skin cancers in this country occur on the face or on the hands and it is first necessary to classify the different types of growth. In rural Ireland most people work in the open air and in such conditions are likely to develop warty growths on the skin. In some cases a wart may develop on the face or hands and grow to be quite large—I have seen one more than an inch high. Normally these are benign but may after some years become malignant.

A more serious condition is called a rodent ulcer. This condition is also likely to occur in people who work out of doors and to appear above a line from the angle of the mouth to the lobe of the ear. It grows slowly and is described as locally malignant, i.e. the growth will invade the neighbouring tissue even eroding bone, but it does not spread to distant parts of the body and if completely removed will not recur.

A still more serious condition is a squamous-celled cancer,

usually called an epethelioma. This is the cancer most usually seen on the lower lip, the face, and in some cases on the hands. An epethelioma will probably spread to the neighbouring glands within a few months.

Now, when a patient consulted a doctor about an unpleasant looking growth on the face or the hand, the doctor could not be sure if the growth was or was not malignant. In order to make sure, he would almost certainly advise the patient to have surgery, or at least to go to a hospital and have a firm diagnosis made. The patient probably answered that he would think over the matter and let the doctor know, and then, with a diagnosis of cancer made by the doctor, he went off. He was then told about all the people who got cured by the cancer curer, so it seemed good sense to get a cancer plaster made. People used to say in County Westmeath:

> the doctor makes the diagnosis and the cancer curer treats the patient.

The essential ingredient in cancer plasters is arsenic. This may be added to lard or butter and applied as a plaster. Sometimes the basis is pitch and I have heard that the juice of ivy leaves is sometimes added. This plaster causes severe pain because the arsenic will destroy all the tissues. It is usual to assure the patient that the more pain the plaster causes, the more surely it is doing the work of killing the cancer. Probably the patient will not get much sleep for a few nights and some people are unable to bear the pain and decide to pull off the plaster. If the patient persists, the pain will get less and after nine or ten days the plaster will probably fall off, and when it does parts of the growth will be found adhering to it. In the only case which I have seen, the resemblance to the claws of a crab (cancer) was striking: I had never understood the reason for the name until I saw this specimen.

The use of arsenic in the treatment of cancer of the skin in modern times was first described in the United States of America by Benjamin Rush. On 3rd February 1786 he read a paper to the American Philosophical Society called 'An Account of the external use of Arsenic in the cure of Cancers'. In his paper, Rush explained that a certain Doctor

Martin of Philadelphia had advertised a cure for skin cancers which he said he had learned from some North American Indians. After the death of Martin, Rush was able to get some of the powder that was used in making the cure, and found that the active ingredient was arsenic. Rush's method was to dissolve the powder in water and paint it on the growth with a feather.

Early in the nineteenth century, a well known Dublin surgeon, Richard Carmichael, wrote a book on his new method of treating cancers. He treated what he said were cases of cancer with different salts of iron. Some of the reports as he presented them seemed impressive, but the patients could not possibly have been suffering from cancer. At the time Carmichael wrote, the diagnosis of cancer could not be made scientifically and if his treatments were successful his diagnoses must have been wrong.

As late as 1887 an escharotic plaster containing arsenic was an official treatment for skin cancer. This is what Whitla of Belfast wrote about it at that time:

> Externally arsenic is a powerful caustic causing the death of the tissue to which it is applied. It is chiefly in cancer and epethelioma that its use has been advocated, but it is dangerous as enough may be absorbed to cause death unless applied in a concentrated form to a very limited extent of surface.

Whitla also gave the composition of what he called Sir Astley Cooper's ointment, which consisted of:

Arsenic   1 dram
Sulphur   1 dram
Make up in Spermacetti to 1 ounce
Sig. Apply the ointment for 24 hours.

There are other preparations which may be used, but none appears to be as effective as arsenic. Sometimes an effort is made by the patient to treat his rodent ulcer or even an epethelioma with caustic soda. This is unfortunate because caustic soda will not destroy all the parts of a malignant growth, and the necessary operation will be made more difficult.

Despite the fears expressed by Whitla, I have never heard of a patient who suffered from arsenic poisoning as a result of the treatment. There was one lady in County Cavan who was famous as a curer of skin cancer. When she died, her funeral was attended by twelve ministers of religion, all of whom were grateful ex-patients and one of whom she had treated for a number of growths over the years.

I have heard of another method used to treat a 'lump' on the lower lip. The lump was rubbed daily with the ashes left in a tobacco pipe. The rubbing was continued for some weeks and ultimately the lump disappeared. It cannot have been cancerous.

Undoubtedly, arsenic plasters could and did destroy certain skin growths. Its best use was the removal of benign growths, and I knew an old man, a relative of mine, who had a dangerous looking wart on his finger removed with an arsenic plaster. The fact that he lost the finger as a result did not shake his faith in the treatment. In the days before anaesthesia was available, the use of arsenic in treating skin growths was a significant advance and until surgery became safer, at the end of the nineteenth century, cancer plasters were as satisfactory as anything else available. It must also be realised that for a considerable time adequate surgery was not available in many parts of Ireland.

The use of cancer plasters appears to have declined in recent years. A few days ago I met a patient from County Longford who showed me the scar of an arsenic plaster on his lip and told me that they are still being used, but, since most of these growths can now be treated by radiation and do not require surgery, it is likely that the use of arsenic plasters will decline further.

I have never heard of any folk treatment for internal cancer. When a cancer curer in County Kerry was asked about this, he answered that the only thing that could cure internal cancer was 'smut éadaigh a bheadh ar chéile sagairt' (a piece of the clothing worn by the wife of a priest). That was his way of saying that there was no cure for the condition.

The use of arsenic in the treatment of skin growths is of more than usual interest. It is a good example of an official remedy which became a folk remedy and was more widely used by folk curers than it ever had been by trained doctors. Like many other such cures, it met a local need and no doubt helped many patients.

CHAPTER III

Bleeding and Wounds

PEOPLE are badly frightened by the sight of blood and, in telling about it, always exaggerate the amount of the bleeding. I remember seeing a pint bottle of blood which was being prepared for transfusion falling and being spilled and I would have sworn that at least four pints had been spilled. Many people have heard of the grave danger of bleeding from an artery and think of this when any bleeding occurs. This greatly adds to their anxiety. The number of treatments used to stop bleeding is very large and generally they have no effect on the bleeding, which will almost always stop no matter what is done. I remember a cut on the sole of the foot which was first treated by tying a necktie around the ankle. This was intended to act as a tourniquet, but in fact it raised the pressure in the veins of the foot and increased the amount of bleeding. When the lady who had the cure arrived, she untied the necktie and the bleeding stopped dramatically.

One treatment with a very ancient and respectable lineage, the application of a cobweb, is still used in every part of Ireland. I do not know how old this treatment is; it is probably as old as the late Latin medical writers of the fourth century and can be found in the Irish translation of the Rosa Anglica. K'eogh knew of this use of the cobweb and wrote:

> The web (of a spider) stops bleeding and prevents inflammation.

Another cure almost equally respectable is the use of the

fur of a hare. A tuft of hair is pulled from the skin, laid directly on the bleeding surface and kept in position with a bandage. K'eogh recommends it and says:

> The hairs or wool (of the hare) are mixed with oint-ments to stop external fluxes of blood.

A fungus with the earthy name of 'bull's fart' (in Irish 'cáise púca') is also used to stop bleeding. It grows in the shape of a ball about five inches in diameter and, seeing it, the metaphor is striking. A more usual name for this fungus is puff-ball (lycoperdon giganteum) and it has long been used in folk medicine to stop bleeding. It has the unusual honour of having been taken from folk medicine and tried out by a Doctor Thompson. This man reported that the dust of the plant, which is largely made up of spores, was a very suitable emergency dressing. He also reported that the dust of the plant sprinkled on a dressing which is plugged into a deep wound will quickly stop the bleeding.

In County Cavan once a young man fell and suffered a severe cut on the hand. It was so severe that the doctor was sent for, but he was not available for some hours. When the doctor got to the patient, he was surprised and perhaps annoyed when he found that the cut had been dressed with a plaster of pig dung. Had the doctor read K'eogh, he might have learned that:

> the dung (of a boar) pulverized, either inwardly taken or outwardly applied, stops fluxes of blood.

Unfortunately, I have been unable to learn if the patient had followed K'eogh's advice fully and taken some of the dung by mouth.

Sugar may be sprinkled on a live coal and the cut finger, or whatever part is cut, held in the smoke from the burning sugar. Butchers, by nature of their work, are liable to cut themselves and have certain methods of their own for stop-ping the bleeding. One of these is to cut off a piece of what they call striffing. This, a thin membrane between the skin and the body fat, is put on the cut and bandaged in place. They sometimes stopped bleeding by rubbing a piece of raw lean meat on the bleeding surface, or they might rub a cut with the raw surface of one of the lymphatic glands which they knew where to find.

The common plantain, in Irish 'copóg Phádraig', is usually referred to in Connacht as 'Saint Patrick's leafeen'. The leaves of this plant are macerated, applied to the wound and covered with a bandage. This treatment is derived from official medicine because K'eogh wrote that plantain was:

> Exceedingly good against haemorrhages and all kinds of fluxes, also useful to conglutinate and heal green wounds.

It was the custom to kill a cock at the feast of Saint Martin (November 11th) and sprinkle the blood at the door. Some of the blood was allowed to fall on a cloth which was then put carefully up in the rafters. This was used to stop bleeding and treat wounds. Bleeding is also stopped by saying some prayers over the wound. One family, living near Poulaphouca in County Wicklow, has the cure which was given to the grandfather of the present holder by a certain Father Heffernan. I understand that words used were a prayer to stop the blood, but I could not learn the exact words —these were a family secret.

Wounds might also be treated with a dressing of unsalted butter; and here is a very genuine folk cure—the person making the cure must chew sorrel (poor man's herb) and spit it on the wound.

The most common source of bleeding, and usually the simplest to treat, is a nose bleed. As children are usually the sufferers, it is important to use a certain amount of ritual and, as in the case of nettle stings, the necessary delay in finding the treatment is important. The best known treatment is to get the largest and coldest iron key possible and put it down the back of the patient's neck. Everybody believed that this was a specific cure. A cold stone, or a cold piece of iron, might be held to the patient's forehead if no key were available. Another method was to put the patient lying flat on his back with his head backwards while grasping the nose tightly and pressing the sides together. This might be a dangerous procedure. The blood would tend to flow backwards into the pharynx and might be inhaled into the lungs. Another method, which seems to be the opposite of the preceding one, was to sit up, lean the head forward and blow the nose vigorously. Plugging the nose would seem to be the obvious method of treatment of a nose bleed, but I have not heard that it was used as a folk cure.

When the bleeding had stopped, it was necessary to dress the wound. One method was to get a piece of strong linen large enough to cover the wound and extending at least a quarter of an inch on to the intact skin. The linen was covered with soft cobbler's wax and applied to the wound. The wax will stick to the skin and form a neat dressing, and in addition it will probably relieve the pain. Unfortunately, it is a most unsatisfactory dressing. After a few days, the surrounding skin will have become soft, white and wrinkled and the wax will have greatly interfered with the natural process of healing. When the dressing was finally removed, the wound was often found to be a dirty mess and when it finally heals there is likely to be a large puckered scar.

I tried to improve on this method by placing a small piece of gauze on the wound and then spreading the wax so that it did not come in contact with the wounded area. Even so, the method is unsatisfactory.

Fresh wounds were often sprinkled with salt. This was quite painful, but the sufferer was consoled when he learned that the greater the pain, the more effectively the salt was working. Formerly, wounds were dressed with carbolic acid solution, or Jeyes' fluid, but this practice has been completely given up. The use of the carbolic acid began about 1880 as part of Lister's antiseptic ritual, when people thought of germs as always harmful. Although this belief is still not quite dead, the damage done by the carbolic acid caused it to be given up. I heard of one case where a carbolic acid dressing to an index finger caused the loss of the finger.

Some wounds needed special care and attention. One of these was a dog bite. I have heard of the wounds being cauterized, but I doubt if this was ever a common practice in Ireland, certainly not for more than fifty years. The usual dressing was with salt, to which a hair of the dog was added. In other cases the hair of the dog was rubbed directly on the wound.

The treatment of a wound caused by standing on a four-pronged fork is of some interest. As this type of fork is normally used for forking dung, it could possibly cause some infection in the wound and people were afraid of this. The type of dressing for the wound is not mentioned, but it was very necessary that the prong of the fork be heated to red heat. This is an example of what is called sympathetic magic. A similar procedure was to heat a sword which had caused a wound.

Wounds were sometimes dressed with a moss found growing on human skulls which had been left exposed to the air. There are many historical references to the use of this moss, usnea cranii humani, to give it its Latin name. After the Confederate Wars, the moss was sent to England on a number of occasions and during the early years of the eighteenth century the skulls of those killed at the Battle of Aughrim were also exported for the moss which was found growing on them.

CHAPTER IV

Fractures

THE sight of an arm or of a leg twisted out of shape following a fracture or dislocation makes a dramatic picture. It is one which most people have seen once or twice and when once seen is never likely to be forgotten. The reduction of the fracture is almost equally dramatic and, when carried out with skill, the relief given to the patient when the operation is completed is satisfactory to everybody. The onlookers, as well as the patient, will be impressed.

Bone-setting appears to have been part of the ordinary leech lore of the mediaeval Irish. Some of the doctors may have specialised in the treatment of fractures and other bone and joint injuries—the Irish surname Mac Cnaimhsi (MacNevin, Kneafsey, Bonar) would suggest this—but there is little direct evidence. Whether this was so or not, there is no doubt that ever since the old Irish period, broken bones were treated efficiently in Ireland and there is a number of references to such treatments in the native annals.

A medico-legal tract called Bretha Déin Chécht has been edited and translated by Professor D. A. Binchy. The basic text is written in the Irish of the eighth century and the manuscript in which it is found, Phillips No. 10297, now G.11, in the National Library of Ireland was written in the fifteenth century. In Section 2B of the text there is a list of the seven most important bone breakings. These were:

1) Tooth. 2) The bone of the arm. 3) The forearm. 4) The thigh bone. 5) The shin bone. 6) The collar bone (delgna gualann, the pin of the shoulder). 7) One

of the bones of the forearm. 8) The pin of the heel (sáldelga).

This last fracture appears to be what is called 'Pott's fracture' of the lower end of the smaller of the two bones of the leg.

These are the most common fractures and also those most easily recognised clinically. In nearly all such cases the diagnosis is obvious and they must have been recognised for thousands of years. The reference to the fracture of one of the bones of the forearm is of interest. This is usually caused by a fall on the outstretched hand, breaking the radius—the lateral of the two bones—just above the wrist, and was classically described by Abraham Colles of Doctor Stevens' Hospital, Dublin, in the Edinburgh Medical Journal in October 1814.

The Lectures of Abraham Colles were published in Philadelphia in 1845. It is notable that in dealing with fractures Colles has not much more to teach than is given more concisely in the Bretha Déin Chécht.

These two references, one from the eighth century and the other from the nineteenth century, give us the basis against which to examine the practice of bone-setting as a branch of Irish folk medicine. Until the development of radiology and antiseptic surgery, the treatment of fractures could not develop and any progress made must depend on the clinical skill of the operator.

Archaeology has been of some help in learning about the treatment of fractures in early mediaeval Ireland. Following the excavation of part of a tenth century graveyard near Castleknock in 1950, the bones of some 380 individuals were examined. Two male collar bones had been broken and in both cases the fractures had united—in one case the union was perfect. Crushed finger bones had also healed in good position.

Before the break-up of the native Irish social system early in the seventeenth century, it is likely that bone and joint injuries were treated by the Irish trained doctor. With the destruction of the native medical schools, it was no longer possible to train doctors, so the art continued as folk medicine. It is easy to speculate that some Irish trained doctor

with special interest, or special skill, in the treating of bone
or joint injuries might teach the art to his son. In the days
before x-rays, the skill that came with long experience and
sound clinical judgement could be acquired by working with
a skilled bone-setter. Compared with this, the training of
an eighteenth century or nineteenth century doctor was very
inadequate. Only during the last quarter of the nineteenth
century was it possible to study the treatment of fractures
scientifically in the Liverpool School of Medicine under
Hugh Owen Thomas, himself the son of a Welsh bone-
setter.

All good bone-setters are familiar with the classical rules:

1) Extension and counter extension
2) Co-aptation
3) Fixation

The first of these, extension and counter-extension, was
often quite difficult because the muscles go into spasm and
when the fracture is some hours old swelling around the
site of the injury will have developed. One of the great skills
of the bone-setter was his ability to pull the fragments apart
without causing much pain to the patient—most of them
did this very skilfully. The counter extension in some cases
was carried out by an assistant or, as in the case of a fracture
of the wrist, by a strong bandage above the flexed elbow and
tied to a hook in the wall. One method used to reduce a
fracture of the shaft of the humerus (arm bone) was to seat
the patient on one side of a half-door with his arm over the
top of the door and hanging down on the other side. A firm
pad was placed on the top of the door to protect the patient's
axilla. The operator could then exert a steady pull on the
arm, so separating the two fragments without much pain to
the patient.

I have heard of this method being used to reduce a dislocation of the shoulder joint. The more usual method, however, which was used by the bone-setter was what is called
the Hippocratic method. In this case the patient's shirt is
removed and he is placed on a firm couch or on the floor.
In case of a dislocation of the right shoulder joint the operator removes his own right boot and, lying alongside the

patient, places his heel in the patient's arm pit (axilla). He then grasps the patient's right hand and, while pressing his heel firmly in the arm pit of the patient, he exerts a steady pull on the arm. This is an efficient method of reducing a dislocation of the shoulder joint.

In treating fractures around the ankles, the patient is seated on a high table with his legs hanging over the edge. Sitting on a low stool, the operator is able to draw the fragments apart. In the case of a very powerful man, the patient may be laid flat on his back on the floor, the thigh is flexed and, while an assistant exerts counter traction on the thigh above the flexed knee joint, the operator is able to separate the broken ends of the bone.

When the bone fragments have been separated, it is then necessary to replace them so as to restore the original line of the bone. This is often a matter of great skill and only long experience can enable the bone-setter to know when he has done it properly.

The method used by the bone-setter to hold the fragments in position is of considerable interest. Before plaster of Paris was available to make splints, many types of splint made of wood and metal were used. When the bone-setter had reduced the fracture, he then decided what type of plaster he should use. If there was much swelling, a light temporary plaster was put on and left in position until the swelling had gone down—in about ten days. This plaster was made of very fine soot mixed with egg white. Bandages were soaked in this and used to make the plaster. A well known bone-setter, the late Patrick Holmes of Ballycastle, County Mayo, used a plaster of flour and egg white. The plaster was smoother than that made with soot and it would probably set firmer. When the swelling had gone down, the plaster was removed and the skin treated with a decoction of comfrey root. This plaster of flour and egg white was used by an English bone-setter to splint a fractured arm of William Cheselden about the year 1700. Cheselden became a famous surgeon and used the plaster in his own practice.

The permanent plaster was made of Burgundy pitch, five parts, and a hard resin called dragon's blood, one part ('sanguis draconis' in the old Pharmacopoeias). These were heated and mixed and, while still soft, the mixture was put over the area of the fracture. The mixture was strengthened by pieces of sacking just as the cotton bandages are used with plaster of Paris. Before the introduction of plaster of Paris, pitch and dragon's blood was a most efficient splinting material available. In some cases it caused considerable irritation of the skin and it was difficult to get off, but in many cases the pitch acted as a counter irritant and relieved the pain.

A major problem of the bone-setter was a fracture of the shaft of the thigh bone, especially a fracture in the upper half of the shaft. In such a case, the upper fragment is flexed by the muscles attached to it, causing great displacement. Added to this, the muscle mass of the thigh makes manipulation very difficult; even if the broken ends are got together, it is difficult to keep them in place. Such fractures still present difficulties even for the most skilful using the most sophisticated equipment.

Dislocation of the head of the thigh bone was also a major problem. Here speed was essential. If the patient is laid on his back on the floor, the dislocation may be reduced by the operator grasping the foot on the affected side while standing on a table and steadily pulling upwards and outwards. The counter-traction is exerted by the patient's weight and his hips may be held flat by an assistant. In this way the displaced head of the thigh bone, which is usually above the socket on the back of the hip bone, is drawn downwards and manoeuvred back into position. In other cases the dislocated bone was replaced by the standard method of flexing the thigh, bending it outwards and rotating it outwards when the head of the bone slipped back into its socket.

Some years ago, tuberculosis of the bones and joints was common in children. In most of these cases the patient gave a history of injury followed by pain in the limb. If a bone-setter was consulted, any manipulation of the diseased joint was certain to do further damage and in one case caused the death of the patient. In fairness to the bone-setter, it must be said that tuberculosis of bones and joints is not an old disease in Ireland and at the beginning people were not aware of the danger. Many bone-setters became aware of the danger and were able to distinguish between tuberculosis and injury.

Bone-setting in Ireland was an hereditary skill. In the area of south Leitrim there were two very well known bone-setters, James Teague and Patrick Donaghy. Both these men had learned the craft from their fathers and the Donaghys had a family tradition that their ancestor was given the power to set bones by Saint Columcille. Some pages of a famous Irish manuscript, the Liber Hymnorum, are preserved in the Franciscan Library, Killiney. A note on one of the pages reads:

> Beandacht o Domhnall mac Dabóg mic Mael Tuili les in leabharsa, et Ase Colam Cill do cur re leghes iat fein a cath Cuildreimne et o Maeltuli Mac Mael Fiath (righ) atait clann mic Mael Tuili i.i slicth Neil nai ngialaigh. Finit.
> (A blessing from Domnail son of Dabhog Mac Mael Tuile to this book and it was Columcille who put them to (practice) medicine at the battle of Cooldreimhne and from Maeltuile son of Mael Fith (ausa) the Clann Mic Mael Tuile is (descended), i.e. they are descended from Nial of the Nine Hostages. The end.)

This family, Mac Mael Tuile (anglicé Tully or Flood) was a well known medical family and practised in the area of Cavan, Leitrim and Longford between 1400 A.D. and 1600 A.D. It may well be that the present Leitrim family is descended from some Mac Mael Tuile, because this entry is not given in the printed edition of the Liber Hymnorum and seems to be a genuine family tradition.

There is a reference to a member of this family who practised surgery in Dublin during the sixteenth century. The man, William O'Moltollye, was arrested by the Members of the Barber Surgeons' Guild in 1572 and again in 1578 and charged with practising surgery while not a Member of the Guild. As he was not 'of English nation', he could hardly have served his apprenticeship and was not eligible for membership of the Guild. In 1578 the charges against him were set out in detail. One of these was:

Said William had one John Tallon his wife in hands
of a broken leg, and did set it crooked and spoiled said
Tallon's wife that she was never able to do herself no
good 'til she died.

This man was almost certainly a member of the Irish medical
family and had got his training in a native Irish school. Unfortunately, there are no further details so we cannot judge
O'Moltollye's skill, or lack of it.

In the neighbourhood of Newmarket in County Cork
there was a well known family of bone-setters called Lane.
One man called Lane had a national reputation, but all the
Newmarket family was well known for its skill in the art.
The O'Leighins were distinguished as a family of scribes
and medical men in many parts of County Cork during the
fifteenth and sixteenth centuries. Here is a colophon of a
section of an Irish medical manuscript, Harley 546, in the
British Museum Library:

Here ends Gualterus, his book of the Doses of Medicine.
Cormac Mac Donleavy it is that for Diarmaid son of
Domhnail O'Leighin has put this summary into Irish
and to himself and sons may so profitable a commentary
render good service. On the 4th day of the Kalends of
April this lecture was finished at Cloyne in the year
when the Lord's annals was 1459.

Many members of this family practise medicine with distinction today, but it also is of interest to see another branch
practising the art of bone-setting.

Clare is a county famous for its bone-setters. The best
known of these were Joseph Sexton and Patrick Burke, both
of whom had represented Clare in the Irish Dáil. Both men
are now dead.

In speaking about bone-setting, people usually stress the
fact that it is an hereditary skill; the bone-setter learned from
his father and in turn taught the art to his son. This is
undoubtedly true, but the names of the bone-setters do not
indicate that the bone-setters of the twentieth century are
direct descendants of the mediaeval Irish medical families.
One notable exception—the Lane bone-setters—has been
mentioned.

Now, bone-setting is unlike most other branches of medicine, either folk medicine or official medicine. In dealing with fractures and dislocations, something positive must be done and the result, favourable or otherwise, will depend to a great extent on the skill of the practitioner. In some other branches of medicine, the patient is likely to get better no matter what treatment is given.

There was always need for a bone-setter. People fell off carts and off horses and off trees, and broke legs, wrists and collar bones. These must be treated efficiently, otherwise people may suffer permanent disability, so it is a social necessity that somebody undertake the work. Patrick Holmes, of Ballycastle, County Mayo, had seen his father treating fractures, but did not himself wish to practise the art. However, there was no other bone-setter available in the neighbourhood and he was almost forced to continue to set bones. From this man's nephew, my friend Doctor Patrick Holmes, I was able to learn an interesting point:

> If you have reduced the fracture and the patient still complains of pain, the fracture is not properly reduced. You must do it again and you must not put on any splint until he is free from pain.

In County Galway I made some enquiries about bone-setting. I learned of a tradition that herds often treated fractures and other injuries in their sheep, calves and pigs and some of them became so skilful that they were called upon to treat their neighbours. I met one man in County Galway who injured his back and was treated by a herd bone-setter with a plaster of Burgundy pitch. He described the treatment by saying:

> It was cruel but good.

There was also an old weaver in north Galway who practised bone-setting with some success.

The Actons were a famous family of bone-setters in the Galway-Mayo border area. Their family tradition is that they came to the district originally as millers but they must have been practising as bone-setters for at least five generations because another family of Actons, rather distant cousins of the present bone-setter, live in the neighbourhood and some members of this family also practised bone-setting many years ago.

I was able to meet the present head of the family, Mr. Tom Acton of Tuam, and he spoke frankly to me about his art. He did not know how long the Actons had been practising, but said that it was more than five generations: he was able to give his genealogy to prove it. I asked if it was thought unlucky for the bone-setter to practise and he agreed that some people said it was. Their cattle were likely to die, people said, but then he added:

People often say that curing disease is unlucky.

We then got down to direct questions. He told me that years ago, following an epidemic of poliomyelitis in County Mayo, he had often been asked to treat some of the patients who had residual paralysis, but he quickly realised that he could not do anything for them:

There was nothing wrong with their bones.

My next question was about tuberculosis of the bones and joints and I was anxious to know how he was able to distinguish between a child with an injured knee and a child with tuberculosis of the knee. He thought about that for a few moments and answered:

Sometimes it's hard to tell. A child with a broken knee is in pain and is likely to be shouting and crying, but he is not a sick child. A child with a T.B. knee is a sick child.

We then spoke of dislocations of the shoulder joint and of the hip joint. He knew exactly the problem in the case of a dislocated hip and was able to demonstrate the method of replacing the head of the thigh bone in the socket. In speaking of dislocations of the shoulder, he distinguished between having the shoulder 'out' and having the shoulder 'down'. This distinction is of importance; it indicates the position of the displaced head of the bone of the arm. If the head of the arm bone was displaced downwards, he used the Hippocratic method by placing his heel in the axilla and pulling the arm. When the bone was 'out', i.e. lying on the back of the shoulder blade, he used the method which was described by Kocher of manipulating the head back into the socket.

I then asked about the danger of a fracture dislocation of the arm bone. Mr. Acton was too polite to say that my question was foolish. Instead he answered:

> You'd have to examine the man and if you weren't sure you could measure the bone.

In treating fractures, his summary was:

> You pull, put the bits together and splint.

That is a good way of saying:

> Extension and counter-extension; coaptation and fixation.

When we spoke of splinting material he said that he used to use a pitch plaster but he preferred an ordinary wooden splint. I asked why and he explained:

> When you put on a pitch plaster it is very hard to get it off again and you cannot judge how the job is going. I like to have a look at it in a week or so.

He then demonstrated on me how he used two flat padded boards on the forearm and tied them together with bows of wide tape, making sure that the knots were on the back splint. He was then able to untie the bows, lift off the back splint and examine the bones without causing pain and with no danger of disturbing the broken ends.

There was not much point in asking any more questions, but I did ask about his use of Burgundy pitch. He told me that a plaster of pitch was very good for a painful back or a painful joint and he used it for such conditions. In these cases the plaster would act as a counter irritant and relieve the pains and aches.

I will end with two expressions which I heard in County Galway:

> The gristle will grow in the bed.

I understand this to mean that the fracture must be reduced

quickly and the patient got out of bed, otherwise the fracture will not unite properly and the patient will have gristle instead of bone. The other expression was:

> The marrow will bung the holeen (fracture), i.e. the marrow will heal the broken bone.

These two expressions show what popular opinion was about the treatment of fractures.

Clearly, the bone-setters provided a necessary service in Ireland. They acquired considerable skill in their art and very few of them made any money from their practice. There was a custom in west Mayo that, if one came for the bone-setter, the messenger stayed and worked for the bone-setter while he was attending the case. There was also the story of the bone-setter who had a habit of calling on his grateful patients long after their treatment had been completed.

Bone-setting in Ireland probably has always been practised by men who did not have formal training in medicine. It is unlikely that a member of one of the recognised native medical families—an O'Hickey or an O'Shiel, for example— would be called to treat a fractured leg bone in a cow herd; no cow herd could afford to pay the fees expected by such men. The regularly trained doctors confined their practice to the aristocracy, and fractures among the common people were probably treated by the bone-setter. In this, the advantage would probably be with the common people.

CHAPTER V

Burns and Scalds

IN this country when a few hot days occur sunburn can be a problem. One might judge this by the number of sunburn lotions, creams and ointments that are advertised and sold. The folk remedies are simple and easily available. The most usual treatment is cream. Sometimes if unsalted butter is available it is used for more extensive burning. In very severe cases, a mixture of buttermilk and bread soda is used. If the curds of the buttermilk are thick and can be separated, they are applied, with the soda, as a compress.

There are many folk remedies for burns and scalds, most of them very useful. Perhaps the best of these is a mixture of one part of bees' wax, by weight, and four parts of mutton fat. The fat must first be boiled and the strings of fibrous tissue removed. The ingredients are then heated together in a double saucepan and stirred until they are blended smoothly. In some cases camomile flowers are added to the mixture, but in my opinion the plaster is better without them. The mixture will remain fresh for months and, when required, some may be taken, heated and applied as a thick dressing to the burn. A better method is to soak linen bandages in the soft mixture while it is being prepared and then these are allowed to harden and are kept until required. When required, the burn is covered with two thicknesses, or more, of the prepared plaster and finished with a bandage to keep the plaster in place. The dressing must not be disturbed for nine days. When it is removed, if the burn has not completely healed the dressing may be repeated.

This is an excellent treatment for a burn and it is stressed that the plaster must be put on as soon as possible after the burn has happened. The heat of the body softens the plaster, which fits snugly to the skin and forms an airtight seal so that the amount of secondary infection of the burned area is greatly reduced. Unless there was a great delay in getting the plaster, or if the burn had been infected by some other form of treatment, healing was likely to be quick and satisfactory. The high melting point of mutton fat is important. If pork fat or beef fat were used, the dressing would soon become a soft mess. The essential points are the quick dressing, the airtight seal and the fact that the dressing must not be disturbed for nine days, because the burn would surely become infected when the dressing was changed.

This method of using a closed dressing anticipated modern surgical practice by at least fifty years, if not much longer. It has been used in exactly this way in County Leitrim for over a hundred years—since my grandmother learned it from her mother. A similar form of treatment was also used in County Wicklow.

The Anglo-Saxon leechbooks have some similar treatments for burns. One of the treatments mentions the leaves of certain herbs and adds the instructions:

boil in butter.

or, better still,

boil in sheep's grease.

In contrast to that method of treating a burn, here is what K'eogh wrote:

An ointment made of it (camomile) with fresh butter and goose dung is an excellent remedy for a burn or scald.

Whatever one may think of this prescription, the essential point has been missed: there is nothing said about a closed dressing and secondary infection would be certain in these cases.

A very primitive form of treatment is to lick the burn. In some cases a dog may be got to do this, but the licking is usually done by the man with the cure. I was able to learn how the power to cure burns by licking them was acquired in County Offaly. Someone who has the power finds someone to whom he wishes to leave the cure and tells him how to acquire it. He is told to go to a certain distance down the road and he will see an alp luachra come out of the rushes on the side of the road. He must pick up the animal, lick its back nine times and put it down on the ground, when it will run into the rushes. The person wishing to acquire the cure must repeat this on nine successive days and when on the ninth day he replaced the alp on the ground it turned over and died. When he returned to the same spot on the following day the alp luachra had gone and in this way he knew that he had acquired the cure. If it had been still there that would show that he was not going to get the cure. The animal called the alp luachra is the common water newt, which is one of the few reptiles found in Ireland.

It is worth recording that the alp luachra had a moment of glory in the history of Irish medicine. It was used by Thomas Molyneux to demonstrate the circulation of the blood before the members of the Dublin Philosophical Society on the 26th of May 1684. This was probably the first demonstration of the circulation in a reptile.

Some other animals may also be licked to acquire the power to heal burns. In some cases a frog may be licked, or a leech. In all these cases the explanation is that the tongue of the licker has acquired a poison from the animal and this poison is able to overcome and drive out the poison that is in the burn.

The ability to acquire healing power from a lower animal is also mentioned in Anglo-Saxon medicine. Here is a quotation from one of the Saxon leechbooks:

> When thou seest a dung beetle in the earth throwing up, grasp him with thy two hands along with his casting, wave him vigorously with thy hands and say thrice 'Remedium facio, ad ventris dolorem.' Then throw the beetle away over thy back. Take care thou look not after it.

The man who had done this had acquired the power to stop:

> Belly-ache in others for the next twelve months by the grasp of his hands.

After these exotic methods, most of the other methods are very ordinary. An emergency method is to add four tea-spoonsful of baking soda to half a pint of thick buttermilk.

The mixture is poured on the burned area, which is then covered with a bandage. I have heard of an extreme case of the use of this method. A badly burned child was taken and plunged, clothes and all, into the churn full of buttermilk. The result was very satisfactory. Probably the buttermilk would relieve the pain. Less elegantly, the fresh urine of a mare, or of a cow, could be used as an emergency treatment. The salt in the urine would probably cause some pain, but if the urine were fresh it probably would be of benefit because it would wash away any dirt which was present and, as fresh urine is sterile, it would not cause any infection of the burned area.

The burn might be dressed with a poultice of egg white. This, when applied to a burn or scald, would probably give some protection if it could be left undisturbed, but this would be unlikely. Another dressing was a mixture of butter and egg yolk, but this again would be very soft and messy.

Scalds were sometimes treated with a preparation of friar's balsam and linseed oil. Friar's balsam was used to protect fresh wounds, and linseed oil was an official treatment for burns. The mixture was quite a good combination in terms of the medicine of the early twentieth century. It would soothe the painful area and in addition it had slight antiseptic action, so it probably would do good.

There is a preparation used in County Clare to treat burns called carron oil. This is the name of an official preparation and the County Clare formula is the same as the official one. The official preparation consisted of lime water 2 ounces; olive oil 2 ounces and the white of 3 eggs. The carron oil was a messy dressing and now appears to have ceased to be a folk remedy.

I have seen a burn treated with a plaster of cow dung. The person making this preparation, if she were asked about its value as a treatment, might have quoted the authority of John K'eogh:

> The dung (of a cow) is proper to be applied to inflammations, phlegmous, or hot tumours, the hot gout, parts burnt, and stung by bees and wasps.

Another old form of treatment for a burn was a poultice of fresh green cabbage leaves, macerated thoroughly and applied along with its juice to the burn. Cabbage is a very old dressing for many things, sore legs, ulcers, and wounds, as well as burns, and is recommended in all the mediaeval text books.

Another treatment for burns is a saturated solution of picric acid, which may still be used in County Meath. Picric acid has been used for a number of things in medicine, including the treatment of burns. It is no longer used officially and probably is now little used as a folk remedy anywhere.

The first snow of the year is sometimes collected carefully and the water is kept. It is used to treat scalds.

Another old method says that a crane should be buried in a manure heap for a month with the bird in a wide-necked suitable container. At the end of the month, some oil will have gathered in the container. This oil is used to treat a burn.

The treatment of burns in Irish folk medicine might be used to illustrate the different parts which go to make it up. There are examples of primitive pagan magic with no pretence of making it a Christian charm. Some of it is derived from mediaeval medicine and there are forms of treatment which are derived from official medicine of the nineteenth century. It will also be noticed that folk medicine, like official medicine, tends to discard forms of treatment when something more efficient becomes available. Most interesting, there is a form of treatment which anticipated the modern treatment of burns by many years.

CHAPTER VI

Boils and Ulcers

BOILS

Boils appear to have been common among the Irish, if we are to judge by the number of folk remedies which were used for their treatment. Before antibiotics were available, a boil could be a very serious condition and a boil on the face could cause death. Similarly, there were many slow, indolent ulcers, most often on the legs, caused by poor circulation of the blood, and also due to chronic infection in a wound.

In the early stages of the infection, a boil is very painful and in severe cases the patient is very ill. The condition may be made much worse by the efforts of the patient, or of his friends, to squeeze the boil in the hope of bursting it. At this stage, squeezing is much more likely to make the condition worse. The natural defences of the body are striving to localise the infection and the squeezing will break down the defences and spread the infection into healthy tissue.

In folk medicine the boil is normally treated with a poultice of some sort. A very popular one was made of soap and sugar. This may have been derived from an official preparation called mel saponis (honey of soap), which I think has now been banished from the pharmacopoeia. This is believed to have great 'drawing' power and is also used to get out a thorn, as well as pus. Until fairly recent times, honey was used as a dressing to protect boils and excoriations.

Another poultice is called in Irish the 'císte uachtair' (cream cake) and comes from County Kerry. It is made of brown flour, brewers' yeast and cream and the preparation is baked as a cake. This is then softened and applied as a poultice to the area of the boil and is said to be quite effective. Still another may be made of the mould of a dried cow pad. The manure is softened in hot water and applied. In the townland of Curradrish in County Mayo a fine clay is found which seems to be kaolin. Poultices for boils or old ulcers are made from this clay and people come many miles to collect it. A simple form of the 'císte uachtair' is made by using a poultice made of ordinary bread. Sometimes Epsom salts were added to the bread poultice. Bread crumb, described under the Latin name of 'mica panis', was employed by official medicine as:

> a soothing application, in the form of a poultice to local inflammations, as it absorbs and retains a considerable quantity of hot water.

These poultices were very comforting to the patient. He felt that something was being done for him and consequently he felt much better. If the poultice was put on early in the infection, it served one very useful purpose: the patient was unable to squeeze the painful area and the bandage holding the poultice was usually large and acted as a splint on the part. This would help to localise the infection.

Surgery, even under the best conditions, is unpleasant and without any form of anaesthetic is very much worse. Most of the poultices would, it was hoped, cause the boil to burst, so avoiding any surgical interference. An ingenious method of bursting the boil has been used in many parts of Ireland. A bottle with a suitably wide neck—a milk bottle—is heated carefully by putting it in water and bringing the water to the boil. It is then taken and the mouth of the bottle is applied to the skin over the boil. As the bottle cools, the air pressure inside falls and the boil is sucked into the bottle. If the skin had become thinned out and weak, it was likely to burst and all was well, but if applied too early in the course of the infection, this might be spread further by the manipulation.

Many of these treatments have an official air about them. The kaolin poultice and the dressing with Epsom salts may have been recently taken over by folk medicine. A patent preparation of kaolin was very widely used up to about twenty years ago and may still be used. When I was a student, a dressing with a solution of Epsom salts was standard treatment for a boil. Even the method of bursting a boil may once have been official: it could be done quite efficiently with a cupping glass.

There is one poultice which appears to be derived from Irish mediaeval medicine. This is called 'the herb poultice' and it is used to dress an infected tendon sheath on a finger (a whitlow) as well as to dress a boil. The herb poultice consisted of the leaves of yarrow, fresh grass and a herb called finabawn. The herbs, equal parts of each, are ground up thoroughly and then beaten up with white of egg. This is put on the inflamed area and must not be changed for forty-eight hours. A whitlow may also be treated by pouring the water in which potatoes have been boiled over the infected finger. The heat from the warm water probably does some good for the condition, but in one case the person pouring on the water was careless, or over-enthusiastic, and the patient got a scalded finger in addition to her whitlow.

There are some additional points of treatment. When one boil occurs, they tend to recur in the same area of skin —the back of the neck was one area where the recurrence was most likely—and it was said in County Leitrim that they would continue until the unfortunate patient had had nine boils in succession. This was prevented by shaving the hairs around the boil and cleaning the area with soft soap and water; as an additional help, the skin might be rubbed with alcohol every day. The only treatment given by mouth of which I have heard was a spoonful of brewers' yeast twice daily.

Fishermen in Newfoundland suffer from crops of small boils on the wrists. These are due to the rubbing of the ends of the sleeves of their oilskins on the skin in very wet, cold weather. In order to prevent these, the men wear about five or six small brass chains on their wrists which impeded the chaffing. This seems to be the correct reason for wearing the chains, although the wearers believed that it was the verdigris of the chains which prevented the boils. Irish fisher-

men do not wear chains, but their weather is not so cold and
I don't think they wear oilskins as much as the Newfound-
landers. I remember a number of cases of men working
under very wet conditions getting crops of boils on their
necks from chaffing of the neck by the oilskins. Their habit
was to use a large silk handkerchief tied neatly around the
neck and they believed that this helped to prevent the boils.

ULCERS

The word ulcer means any condition which is very slow to
heal. Ulcers may be due to many different conditions, of
which probably the most common is varicose veins. Many
old wounds were heavily infected and perhaps contaminated
with dirt or some other foreign body—a piece of clothing,
for example—which would prevent its healing. Also, the
longer the wound remained unhealed, the more fibrous
tissue formed around it, cutting off the blood supply and so
further interfering with the healing. Many such ulcers were
formerly treated with Jeyes' fluid or even pure carbolic acid,
but these are no longer used in Irish folk medicine.

Varicose ulcers used to be called the opprobrium chirur-
gorum (the reproach of surgeons) because for centuries they
were incurable. This was because official medicine had not
learned the necessity for rest and proper bandaging. In Irish
folk medicine these ulcers have been treated by applying the
yellow head of the ragwort and bandaging it over the site of
the ulcer. Before doing so, the head was dried and reduced
to a powder and this would require a larger and more
efficiently applied bandage than if the head were used fresh.
The use of the ragwort may be derived from K'eogh, who
wrote:

(Ragwort is) a great traumatic, special good to heal
wounds, fistulas and ulcers.

I do not know what effect ragwort would have on an old
ulcer—probably none—but a properly applied bandage from
the toes to below the knee would certainly help to heal the
ulcer.

A 'sore leg' may also be treated with a poultice of dock
leaves. It is first necessary to remove and discard the central

stem of the leaves which are then warmed before the fire and teased out and softened by hand. When the leaves have been thoroughly softened they are applied as a poultice. This poultice was believed to be very useful to clean out pus and get rid of old sloughs, leaving a clean wound.

A similar poultice to treat ulcers was made of cabbage leaves, preferably green leaves. The leaves might be laid flat on the ulcer, but the more usual method was to break up the leaves—a hand mincer has been used—and apply the soft mess as a poultice, which would require a large and firm bandage. Cabbage is a very ancient remedy and is prescribed as a dressing for many conditions in the Rosa Anglica and these include infected swellings and ulcers. The reason for breaking up the leaves may be to release the juice, because K'eogh says:

> All coleworts have much the same virtues. They make the belly soluble, their juice with the meal Fenugreek helps the gout, cleanses and heals old rotten sores.

This use of green leaves of dandelion and cabbage recalls the many uses found some years ago for chlorophyl, the green colouring matter of plants.

A plaster of warm cow dung is also used to treat all sorts of ulcers, more usually varicose ulcers. Here again K'eogh has something to say about the many medicinal uses of cow dung:

> The dung is proper to be applied to inflamations, phlegmous or hot tumours, the hot gout, parts burnt, and stung by bees and wasps. It is Antifebritic, good against burning fevers, and the collic. The juice of it being pressed out and drank it is with success thus made use of by common people for the said disorders.

The broadest spectrum antibiotic could not do anything that cow dung could not do better.

One dramatic cure of an ulcerated hand deserves to be remembered. According to my informant, a patient was admitted to Castlebar Hospital to have an infected hand amputated. While waiting for the operation, he heard of an old woman from the mountains of west Mayo who had the power of curing infected hands, so the patient left hospital and found her. She was eighty years old and said that she was too old for the cure but he persuaded her to try it. She took some blood out of her arm, mixed it with unsalted butter and dressed the hand, which quickly healed. This is another example of blood used to treat different conditions. It is clearly derived from paganism and was forbidden in the Anglo-Saxon Penetentials.

Another dressing for an ulcer was made from a ray. The fish was first boiled for some hours until it was reduced to a jelly which was then applied to the ulcer and bandaged in position. A more modern type of treatment for any old, indolent ulcer was balsam of Peru. This is taken directly from official medicine and this quotation from Whitla may be the source of the cure:

> Externally the Peruvian balsam is a mild stimulating application to sluggish ulcers, bed sores and cracked nipples.

I have been assured by highly intelligent people that many of these treatments have healed old ulcers. Certainly the extensive bandages necessary to hold the poultices in position would be of help, but in the case of a varicose ulcer it would be necessary to keep the patient in bed or at strict rest. The necessity for rest is never mentioned in describing the treatment; the healing powers are all attributed to the material used in the dressing. I have wondered if the people making the poultices realised the necessity for rest but did not wish to have the patient realise this; that would make the cure much too simple. Perhaps the patient was warned about the danger of displacing the bandage and this would be likely to limit his activities.

CHAPTER VII

A Thorn

Dealg láimhe nó focal amadáin.
(A thorn in the hand or the word of a fool.)

THE Irish expression sums up succinctly the discomfort and annoyance caused by a thorn in the hand. In a rural community, when people often went barefoot and hedge cutting was a common occupation, a small splinter under the skin must have been a common accident. In removing it, care must be taken to see that every part has been removed and even today this may be quite difficult. Without any form of anaesthetic and often in the presence of infection, the removal of a thorn must have been painful and distressing for the patient and for his anxious relatives. With no great certainty of success it cannot have been pleasant for the medical attendant either. When the person treating the case did succeed in getting out the thorn, it was a triumph, but in many cases his cutting and probing must have destroyed the efforts by the body to localise the infection which would then spread further.

Some charms to help remove thorns, splinters and such things can be found in old Irish manuscripts. One of these written in old Irish can be found in the Codex Sangallensis. The charm has been translated:

> Nothing is higher than heaven, nothing is deeper than the sea. By the holy words that Christ spoke from his Cross remove from me the thorn . . . Very sharp is Gobniu's science. Let Gobniu's goad go out before Gobniu's goad.

This charm is laid in butter which goes not into water,
and some of it is smeared all round the thorn, and it
(the butter) goes not on the point, nor on the wound,
and if the thorn be not there one of the two teeth in the
front part of his head will fall out.

A modern version of this use of butter is to put unsalted
butter on the skin around where the thorn is supposed to be.

Despite the reference to Christ, the words of this charm
are more pagan than Christian. The first twenty-six words
are probably repeated by the patient, partly as a prayer to
Our Lord and partly as a prayer to Gobniu, the name of some
Irish pagan deity. The name Gobniu would suggest some
iron-worker god. The threatened loss of the two teeth was a
very serious one in old Irish society and a very large amount
of compensation was payable for such an injury. The threat
is much more pagan than Christian in spirit.

Another charm against a thorn has been found in the
Stowe Missal. It is also written in old Irish and has been
translated:

> A splendid salve (macc saele = filius sputi = son of spit)
> which binds a thorn. Let it not be spot or blemish, let
> it not be swelling nor illness, nor clotted gore, nor
> lamentable hole, nor enchantment. The sun's brightness
> heals the swelling, it smites the disease.

This is certainly a pagan charm with its reference to the
sun's brightness healing the disease. The list of complications against which the charm asks for protection shows what
might happen to a person injured by a thorn or splinter. The
meaning of the first few words is not quite clear. I take them
to mean that the wound was anointed with spittle which was,
and still is, used in many folk remedies and remained in the
official Pharmacopoeia until the end of the eighteenth century. The essential point about it is that it is the giving of
something personal by the person making the cure to the
patient. The Codex Sangallensis is of the ninth century and
the Stowe Missal goes back to the seventh century. The words
of the charms may have been written later, but not later
than the eleventh century.

In modern folk medicine a piece of fat bacon might be put on the wounded area and kept in place with a bandage. The salt in the bacon would be likely to irritate the skin, but the bandage would serve a useful purpose. If left undisturbed it would act as a splint, thus immobilising the part and helping to localise the infection and the thorn might be extruded or enclosed with fibrous tissue.

Another popular treatment was a poultice of soap and sugar. This was used when it was clear that the wound had become infected and an abscess was forming. As the abscess developed, the skin became thinned out and pus formed and the abscess was likely to burst and the thorn might be discharged with the pus. Many people have assured me that a poultice of soap and sugar was a very satisfactory method of dealing with the infection caused by a thorn.

I heard of a folk cure for the removal of a thorn which is used in France. A very tiny piece of cobbler's wax is made soft and placed in the hole caused by the thorn and bandaged in place. The wax causes the death of the tissues around the hole, forming a tiny ulcer and preventing the wound from closing. As in the case of the poultice with soap and sugar, the thorn is likely to come out with the pus.

As a doctor in a Canadian logging town, I once had some experience of trying to get out splinters and thorns. These were certainly the commonest accidents which I handled and in dealing with them I was greatly helped by the fact that the woodsmen realised that such accidents could become very difficult.

CHAPTER VIII

Baldness

Physicians of the utmost fame,
Were called at once but when they came
They answered as they took their fees
There is no cure for this disease.

THERE is no need to explain the importance of treatments for baldness. The ordinary type of baldness in the young or youngish male is a source of great anxiety and trouble to the sufferer and he is the one most likely to search hopefully for treatment. A modern book on skin diseases has this to say:

> No treatment has any effect but coexistent seborrhoea capitis, which aggravates the condition, should be treated.

Be that as it may, people have always sought for cures for baldness and will continue to do so.

One form of treatment favoured in County Kerry and County Clare is of interest. Human urine is poured into the bladder of a goat which is then hung up in the chimney above the fire and it must remain there until all the liquid has evaporated. When this has happened, the bladder is taken down, ground up and rubbed on the scalp.

There is another preparation made with worms. The person making it up must fill a jar with worms and bury the jar in the manure heap; at the end of a month the jar may be dug up and the contents rubbed on the scalp.

Treatments similar to these may be found in the mediaeval Irish medical manuscripts. Here are two taken from the Irish translation of the Lilium Medicinae, the original of which was written by Bernard of Gordoun, a famous Professor at Montpellier, about the year 1305:

> Let calcine a raven. His ashes boil in sheep's suet. Rub to the head and it cures.
>
> With mice fill an earthen pipkin. Stop the mouth with a lump of clay and bury beside a fire, but so as the fire's too great heat reach it not. So it be left for a year and at a year's end take out whatsoever may be found therein. But it is urgent that he that lift it have a glove upon his hand lest at his fingers' ends the hair come sprouting out.

I once mentioned this treatment for baldness in a popular article and one reader wrote and asked me for some of the preparation. Another found out where I lived and came looking for some of it. I felt like a prophet getting honour in his own country when I learned that this treatment had become part of the folk medicine of County Leitrim.

After these exotic forms of treatment, the other methods are less interesting. Bone marrow of a cow is sometimes rubbed hopefully on the scalp. Neat foot oil may also be used. This has a slightly irritating effect which might give the patient some hope for a while. I have known one man who went to a barber and had his head shaved completely. Presumably the reason for this was the mistaken belief that shaving stimulates the growth of hair; adolescent males used be advised not to shave for that reason. Blistering the scalp has also been tried and one preparation sold as a treatment for baldness contains enough cantharides to make the scalp red. Another hopeful method is to rub the scalp with a raw onion.

From County Galway I heard of an ointment. The burned embers of a sally tree are ground very fine and mixed with hog's lard and turpentine to form a thick paste. The instruction said:

> Apply the ointment nightly and rub hard;

and, as a saver,

> this is no good if the roots of the hair are dead.

There are two 'hair tonics' which are clearly taken directly from official medicine and have now become folk remedies.

Salicylic acid	80 grains
Bay Rum	3½ ounces
Olive oil	½ ounce
spirit to	8 ounces.

The instructions say that it should be rubbed into the scalp night and morning.

The other is made up as an ointment and is called 'Bear's Grease'. It contains:

Coconut oil	3 ounces
Oil of lemons	10 drops
Oil of Rosemary	20 drops
Tincture of Cantharides	1 dram
Yellow Vaseline to	8 ounces

and so it goes on. There will always be young men who will lose their hair and many of these will look for the cure that has so far not been found; and, if one must tell the unpleasant truth, there is no evidence that any efficient treatment for the ordinary case of baldness will ever be found. In the meantime, boiled mice and rotten worms and other such remedies will give temporary hope to the patients.

CHAPTER IX

Warts in Children

IT may be said that all children get warts. These are due to a virus infection of the skin and usually appear shortly after the child begins to go to school. Sometimes they spread widely on the hands and may be a great source of anxiety to a sensitive child when other children notice and comment on them. The list of cures for these warts appears to be endless—one can always learn of another one—and they are all about equally successful. I do not know to what extent dermatologists treat them, but it seems that the great majority of the sufferers are treated with some folk remedy which is simple, cheap and quite effective.

It seems certain that their success is due to very good psychotherapy, often by people who never heard of psychotherapy and would not believe it if they were told about it. The people who treat and cure warts know that their treatment is successful, they have plenty of evidence to prove it. They may offer different explanations of why their treatments work—the power of a saint, or the healing powers of the skin of a black snail—but the essential point is that the treatments work.

In general there are three forms of psychotherapy. One conveys the idea of wasting, causing the warts to waste away. Another is a symbolic washing, and the third conveys the idea of transferring the warts to someone else. I know of a dramatic example of the wasting idea. The patient was a student nurse in a famous Dublin teaching hospital and her hands were so severely infected that she was not allowed to work in the operating theatre. For some years she had been attending doctors but the warts were still there. If she were not allowed to work in the operating theatre she might be forced to give up nursing, so in her difficulty she consulted the hospital Matron, who was a special friend. The Matron said: 'I will cure you.' She got a piece of raw meat and made the Sign of the Cross with it over each wart, taking care that no wart was missed. When this had been done, she buried the piece of meat in the clay in a large flower pot in her room and explained that as the meat rotted the warts would disappear. When about a week later the Matron enquired about the warts they had all disappeared.

There are many other examples of such wasting cures. The warts may be rubbed with a black snail and the snail is then impaled on a thorn tree. As the snail dries up and withers, the warts also wither and disappear. There is another version of the black snail treatment. The rubbing must be done early in the morning on two Mondays and one Thursday and then the snail is sacrificed on the thorn tree. The piece of meat may be fat bacon and this should be buried in the manure heap. A Dublin version of this method is to rub the warts with the raw surface of a potato, which is then buried in clay. To make perfectly sure, the treatment may be repeated on the following day using the other piece of the potato, or in some cases it may be done a third time. A similar method is to cover the wart with a plaster for about ten days and when the plaster is removed the wart may be found to have disappeared. This method may have been taken over from official medicine, but the others are clearly examples of native magic.

A dramatic wasting cure is used in the neighbourhood of Trim, County Meath. In a ruined church near Newtown Bridge there is a sixteenth century altar tomb with stone figures of a husband and wife on top of it. Water accumulates in a channel around the top of the tomb and a visitor will notice a large number of pins lying in the water in all stages of rustiness. The cure is performed by taking a pin and pointing it at each wart in turn. The pin is then placed in the water and as it rusts away the warts will disappear. I have treated my own children's warts in this way and within a week the warts had gone.

The washing charms are simpler and more widely used. The warts may be treated by dipping them in the water of many holy wells. There is a famous wart well at Clonard (County Meath), the virtues of which are attributed to Saint Finnian. The well is a round shaded hollow of a rock and there is no obvious source of the water in the well. There is a famous wart well near Holywood, County Wicklow, and another at Deisert, near Ballinakill, County Laois. At Mulhuddart in County Dublin, Saint Brigid's well also cures warts, but the water of most holy wells is used and they can be found all over the country. If for any reason the sufferer cannot go to a holy well, he may treat his warts by bathing them in water found in a hollow stone. This is even more effective if he happens to find the water when he is not looking for it.

There is a very famous wart stone in County Leitrim. This is in the townland of Beaghmore, about a mile from the village of Carrigallen. The wart stone is a large rock with a cup-shaped hollow in the top where rain collects. The warts are dipped in the water, but I have not heard of any prayers or other form of ritual.

Another washing cure is to use forge water—the water used by the smith to cool the hot iron. The bathing should be done every morning for nine mornings. Here there is a difficulty. The water must be stolen by someone other than the patient.

The warts may also be treated by rubbing them with fasting spittle, each morning for nine mornings, or until the warts are gone. When I looked to see what K'eogh had to say about the virtues of fasting spit, I learned that it might be used to treat the bite of a mad dog or of a serpent. I have heard of children in Dublin who treated their warts by dipping them in an inkwell at school.

Some examples of cures by transference may now be given. In one such method, the sufferer collects pebbles, one for each wart, and places them at a cross roads. The first person who comes along and picks up the stones will get the warts. Another example of a transference cure is to buy the warts from the patient. I once used this method but not with complete success. However, I am happy to say that the cure was completed by someone more expert than I. As instructed by him, the patients, two very bright young girls, stole a rasher (from their mother), cut off a piece of it for each wart and buried the pieces in the ground. The warts disappeared.

There is a method used in County Clare in which the warts are treated by remote control, as it were. To make the cure, someone, not necessarily the patient, but no doubt with his agreement, must go and tell the curer that so-and-so wishes to be cured of warts and when the curer agrees to cure them that completes the treatment. As far as I could learn, there is no ritual or special prayers, but it seems that it is a case of transferring the warts to the curer.

In addition to all these, there is a miscellaneous group which work equally well. The sufferer may touch the coat of a man who never saw his own father. In addition, he must be careful in doing this that the owner of the coat does not notice him doing it. I knew one man who had a reputation for the successful treatment of warts in this way. He was very careful not to notice children who came near him. One may also tell the sufferer that the warts are likely to spread all over his body. I have not used this unpleasant method, but I have been assured that it has worked well. Two other methods may be of interest. Castor oil applied daily for a week or so has been successful. The milky sap squeezed from the dandelion may also be rubbed on the warts.

Turner (1736) gives a number of treatments for warts. These include the juice of a large number of plants and among these is:

> succus lacteus e caulibus Dentis Leonis
> (the milky juice from the leaves of the dandelion).

In the course of his article on the treatment, he says:

> I shall not stay to enlarge upon some other remedies having little other than direct Foolery or Superstition for their foundation: such as cutting a certain stick with so many notches, the stealing of Beef to rub them with and after burying same in the Earth.

These methods of transferring, washing and wasting warts are probably thousands of years old and such methods are found in Anglo-Saxon magic. I do not know of any ancient

Irish charms to remove warts. This is not surprising; there were many successful treatments, so there was no reason to write one down.

There are many treatments for warts which are derived from mediaeval medicine. A mixture of goat's droppings and unsalted butter is typical of these. There are many such prescriptions found in the Rosa Anglica, probably because, as the author says, he himself suffered from them. One of these is an ointment prepared from ashes of snails mixed with stale unsalted lard. A similar sort of preparation is an ointment made of goat's droppings mixed with vinegar.

As would be expected, K'eogh gives a number of treatments. One of these is:

> Being outwardly applied and well mixed with yellow Clay (the urine of an ass) cures scabs, warts, callous parts and eases the Pain of the gout.
> If that does not work 'The fat (of a bull) mixt with Rue' may be used.

Another method recommended by K'eogh is:

> the Ashes of the Dung (of a calf) mixt with vinegar cures Warts and stops Blood.

One might go on citing more cures, but they all follow the same pattern and would add little to the general picture. It is clear that whatever effect these forms of treatment, from the Rosa Anglica or K'eogh, may have had was due to psychotherapy. It must be admitted that washing with water from a holy well or rubbing with a piece of beef is pleasanter than applying the dung of a goat or a calf. It would seem that the cleaner and more pleasant methods superceded the others in modern Irish folk medicine.

As seems clear, it is possible to remove warts in children by psychotherapy. That being so, it would be expected that drinking or applying the water of spa wells might be used to cure warts. Rutty gives many examples of skin diseases which were so cured but does not mention warts. Perhaps the explanation is that the methods of treating the warts were established before the use of spa water became popular and there was no need for them: the older methods were satisfactory.

Having written this, I looked up the modern treatment of warts in children. The author clearly recognises that warts may disappear and this may be helped by psychotherapy. As treatment, he advises:

destruction by chemical (salicylic acid, Podophyllin or formalin) or physical (burning, freezing or curettage) methods.

There are two causes given for warts in children. One is the belief that they are caused by wetting the hands with the water in which eggs have been boiled. Children are warned that if they pick at a wart and make it bleed, the blood will cause the warts to spread.

CHAPTER X

The Sprain

A SPRAIN is a rather vague diagnosis. In a general way it means an injury in the neighbourhood of a joint without any fracture or dislocation. More precisely, it means a ruptured ligament or tendon, but in folk medicine no very precise definition is necessary or needed. The word may be used to flatter the patient in much the same way as 'a dose of the flu' sounds much more important than a 'cold'; similarly, some patients would be better pleased to be told that they were 'threatened with pneumonia' than to have a mild chest infection shrugged off as of little significance. In County Leitrim a distinction is sometimes made between a strain and a sprain. The strain is the less severe injury.

The simplest form of treatment is to turn the cold tap on it. A more elaborate method is to rub the painful area with grease or unsalted butter. The object here appears to be to massage the painful area and the butter or goose grease would make the massage less painful. Sometimes the patient went to a weaver, who tied a weaver's knot around the painful area. There are other versions of this tying something round the sprain. A string with nine knots may be tied, or a piece of red thread. I do not know why the material should be red, but, as in the case of red flannel, red is the colour used to expel demons.

A standard method was to apply a poultice of comfrey roots. This poultice was also used to ease the pain of any hurt or bruise and as a mild irritant it might well relieve the pain. K'eogh says:

The roots (of comfrey) beaten to a cataplasm give ease to the gout.

There are other herbal remedies for a sprain. A poultice of bog onions may be used in County Clare and I have been assured that such a poultice gives considerable relief. K'eogh had this to say about bog onions:

The root is bulbous and is divided into cloves like garlic. A clove of this put into a glass of water will in half an hour make it very thick and ropy which being put upon a cloth is very good to be applied to luxations and dislocations.

Bog moss is also used to treat a sprain. As the moss is being gathered care must be taken to see that it remains wet from the damp peat in which it grows. The sprained limb is put in some suitable container and the damp moss is packed well around it. Alternatively, if necessary, a thick poultice of the damp moss may be applied to the sprain. K'eogh does not mention bog moss.

There is an interesting method of treating a sprain which I learned in County Leitrim. In this case the person performing the cure places his hands on the painful area and says:

Our Lord was going over the mountain and his foal's foot he sprained. Down he got and touched the sprain and said he: 'Bone to bone, blood to blood, nerve to nerve, and every sinew in its proper place'.

This would seem to be an ordinary narrative charm in which faith healing and a primitive form of laying on hands was used. It is, however, rather more than this. Singer has translated and quoted a charm from a tenth century German manuscript:

Phol and Woden
Fared to a wood
There was Balder's
Foal's foot sprained
· · · · ·
Then charmed Woden

> As well he knew how
> For Bone sprain
> for Blood sprain
> for Limb sprain
> Bone to Bone
> Blood to Blood
> Limb to Limb
> As though they were glued.

John Windle described another version of the sprain charm:

> Christ went on the Cross: a horse's leg was dislocated.
> He joined blood to blood, flesh to flesh, bone to bone.
> As he healed that may he heal this.

It would be interesting to trace the history of this charm. Singer said that versions of it were found in the Highlands of Scotland as well as in different parts of Ireland. Perhaps at the beginning the god invoked was Dian Cécht, the Irish god of healing, or Brigit, the goddess of healing, as Woden was the Norse god.

CHAPTER XI

The Teeth

There is no philosopher however great who could bear the toothache with patience.

THAT quotation has been attributed to Socrates, but whether he said it or not, to nearly everybody it is most painfully true. To many people their earliest memory of pain is the toothache, which followed a gluttonous feed of sugary sweets, so nearly everyone is able to tell of some method of relieving the pain.

In one of the great Irish manuscripts—the Lebor Breac—a charm against toothache is found written in a margin and has been translated by Whitley Stokes. The translation runs:

> May the thumb of chosen Thomas in the side of guilt-less Christ heal my teeth without lamentation from worms and from pangs. Pater noster before and after.

Singer has shown that the idea that worms cause tooth-ache is a part of primitive Anglo-Saxon magic, but this charm shows that the native Irish also believed in worms as a cause of disease. There must be very few people who cannot re-member poking at a painful tooth with their fingers.

There is another narrative charm which I learned from a man from County Westmeath. In telling of the charm his words were exact:

> As Saint Peter sat on a marble stone Our Lord was passing and asked: 'What aileth thee Peter?' Peter answered: 'Lord, my tooth aches'. The Lord said: 'Arise

Peter and be going'. Let this be known to all who say these words. They will not suffer from toothache.

It would seem from the wording that the sufferer said the words after the person performing the cure. Versions of this charm can be found in Anglo-Saxon and Middle English manuscripts and it is also used in Brittany and the Highlands of Scotland.

In my native parish in County Leitrim a sufferer might do a round of the stations in the old graveyard near Ballinamore and at Saint Brigid's well a few fields away. There was a number of special days in the year when this might be done and if the sufferer was too busy or too lazy to do it himself it might be done on his behalf by someone else.

In the days before anaesthesia, the extraction of teeth was a painful and sometimes dangerous undertaking. A dramatic example of the danger can be found in the Calendar of State Papers. On 11th March 1637 the Lord Deputy wrote to his friend Lord Conway telling him the news from Dublin and adding at the end of the letter:

> Sir James Erskine had a tooth drawn the other day. The dentist pulled it out at one clap and also two others which he could have been content to have kept. You may chance to laugh at this but Sir James got a fever from it which killed him two nights ago. I shall like worse of pulling out of teeth for a twelvemonth.

Some forms of treatment were fatalistic. The attitude was that there is no use in trying to do anything if the jaw is greatly swollen. It is necessary to wait for nine days and by that time the acute phase of the infection will have passed. The patient might not be greatly consoled by this advice, but in all the circumstances it was very sound and safe and avoided interference which would almost certainly cause a spread of the infection. Even today it is much wiser to control the infection with a suitable antibiotic before interfering with the offending tooth. He was a wise folk dentist who first gave that advice.

It is not usually difficult to get out the milk teeth in children. When the tooth has been got out, with or without the help and sympathy of his school friends, it must then be disposed of in the recognised way. In County Leitrim the owner of the tooth must throw it over his left shoulder and must not look to see where it went. This is an example of primitive magic in which the tooth and the pain and discomfort which went with it were transferred to the earth. Parents often took care to see that the child did this and, for good measure, told the child that if he did not do it he would not grow any bigger. A slightly more modern version is to put the tooth in a glass of water. This was left overnight for the fairies who left some money in exchange for the tooth.

In some areas the local blacksmith also acted as a tooth puller. When the sufferer consulted him he decided if the tooth should be pulled or not. If he decided to take the tooth out, he tied a strong thread waxed with cobbler's wax around the tooth and tied the other end to the anvil. He then put a piece of iron in the fire, made it red hot, beat it on the anvil, made it red again and suddenly moved as though to jab the red iron in the sufferer's face. The sudden jerk backwards, it was hoped, would pull out the tooth. My father assured me that he had known this method to work, but the tooth must have been quite loose. I have often heard of this method but never happened to see it being done. Probably the blacksmith knew when he examined the tooth that it could be got out in this way.

I have heard often of a famous 'Doctor' Sequa who worked at the fairs of the north midlands as a tooth drawer as well as a seller of his own medicines. As part of his act he travelled in a coach accompanied by a brass band. According to the many stories about him, the band made the necessary amount of noise to drown the shrieks of the patient as the tooth came out.

There were a few forms of treatment to help ease the pain; a plug of cotton wool soaked in oil of cloves has recently moved from official to folk medicine. In Dublin a recognised treatment was to rub mustard on the painful area. The counter-irritation by the mustard might be of considerable benefit. Still another method was to touch the nerve of the tooth with a horseshoe nail. My own toothaches, as a child, were treated with a plug of cotton wool soaked in this mixture:

Liquid carbolic acid	6 drams
Oil of cloves	6 drams
Camphor	$4\frac{1}{2}$ drams
Chloroform	$\frac{1}{2}$ a fluid ounce

The camphor was dissolved in the chloroform and then the other ingredients were added.

TOOTH PASTE

When I was a boy, people had learned the value of brushing the teeth, but tooth paste was rarely used. Fine soot was used and also a mixture of soap and salt, or baking powder and salt.

And to end, here is a cure for neuralgia taken from nineteenth century manuscript, No. 23.G.41 in the Royal Irish Academy. It reads:

> Cure for Neuralgia. Best ever discovered.
> One of Gallen's (?) Recipis (?)
> $\frac{1}{2}$ a dram of sal aminomia (?) in an oz. of camphor water. To be taken, a teaspoonful at a dose. A dose repeated at interval of five minutes if the pain is not removed at once.

The writer of the manuscript was trying to make the most of his cure, which he quite wrongly attributed to Galen.

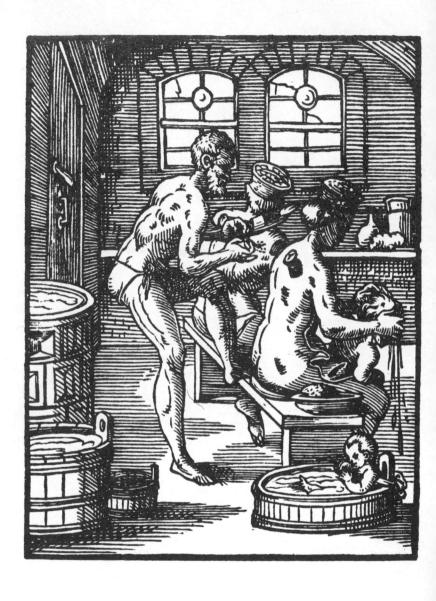

Part 3

Methods of Treatment

CHAPTER I

Holy Wells

THERE are hundreds of holy wells in Ireland. There can scarcely be a parish in the country, outside the bigger cities, which has not at least one and it would require a book much larger than this one to deal with the subject. Some of these wells are visited by people seeking cures for diseases and therefore they may be regarded as a part of Irish folk medicine. While the custom of visiting the wells is generally very old, and in many cases clearly pre-Christian in origin, some of them are comparatively modern. The custom of visiting two famous wells began in the nineteenth century and a more famous one still may have started during the eighteenth century.

As it is impossible to deal adequately with all the wells which are believed to cure diseases in the space of one short chapter, I will describe a few which I believe are typical of the hundreds of such wells in Ireland.

There is a famous holy well, now dedicated to Saint Brigid, near Liscannor in County Clare. The well is visited on the last Sunday of July, which is the traditional date of the end of summer, and was celebrated as the festival of Lughnasa by the pre-Christian Irish. No doubt the custom of visiting the well and the celebration on the strand at Lahinch are pre-Christian survivals, but there is enough evidence around the well to show that it has been thoroughly Christianised. The votive offerings, crutches, holy pictures, rosaries, etc., left inside the well house testify to the faith of the pilgrims and to the belief that diseases are cured there.

The station consists of the recitation of six Our Fathers and six Hail Marys while going around an outer ring of stations. This is repeated six times. A similar round of an inner ring also saying six Our Fathers and six Hail Marys six times and kissing an ancient crucifix is next and the station is completed by drinking some of the water of the well.

In her book on the Festival of Lughnasa, Maire Mac Neil gives the evidence for believing that this began as a pre-Christian festival, but the name of the well in Irish, Dabhach Bhríde (Brigit's Well), would indicate that the baptism of the festival occurred in early Christian times.

At Tarmonbarry in County Roscommon there is a very old graveyard with a ruined church and a holy well nearby. Until a few years ago many people visited the well, prayed there and drank the water. I was told that few people now visit it, but when I was there I saw rags tied on the bushes showing that cures are still being sought and certainly people believe that a visit to the well may cure some diseases.

An unusual power attaches to the ruined church. It is believed that if a patient suffering from a mental illness went with a companion and slept one night in the ruins his illness would be cured. If he went, but did not sleep, the outlook was less favourable. Clearly any patient who had sufficient insight into his condition and was so co-operative as to sleep during the visit was quite likely to have a good prognosis.

On Saint Mogue's Island in Templeport Lake in County Cavan, a station is made every year on 31st January. Those doing the station sometimes bring home clay from the island, but before doing this it is necessary to bring in more clay than the pilgrim intends to bring out. The clay is kept in the home, and has the power of protecting it and everyone in it against harm by fire and by wind. During the 1939-45 war, a woman living in the neighbourhood had a son who was flying with the R.A.F. She sent him some of the clay which he carried with him and his planes always came home safely.

There are many holy wells in the area of south Leitrim and west Cavan dedicated to Saint Patrick and some of them are reputed to cure diseases. The traditional story of their origin is that Saint Patrick, when he had destroyed the idol Crom Cruach on Magh Sléacht near the village of Ballymac-gauran, moved along the east face of Sliabh an Iarainn and round the south shoulder to cross the Shannon. At each place where he rested he preached to the people and healed them and the wells have been visited ever since. Perhaps the best known of these is one in the townland of Miskawn Glebe in the parish of Outeragh. The well is covered by a concrete well house. When I was last there, the path from the road along a small mountain stream was well worn and the bushes around the well were hung with the usual pieces of cloth.

This practice of tying a piece of cloth on a bush near the well is observed in every part of Ireland. Nobody in the neighbourhood of any of the wells was able to suggest any reason why it was done; 'It's always done.' Originally it may have been a votive offering, i.e. leaving a piece of clothing belonging to the patient or to the person seeking the cure on behalf of the patient. In any case it does not seem like a Christian practice in origin.

There was another well dedicated to Saint Patrick on the southern face of Sliabh an Iarainn at a place called Pulty, which is also reputed to cure the usual things, sore eyes, warts, etc. There was a pattern held here on the last Sunday of July, but the well might be visited on any day to obtain a cure.

There is a famous well dedicated to Saint Fechin at Fore in County Westmeath. It can be found near the ruins of the ancient church and is a considerable distance from the mediaeval ruins of the Benedictine Priory. There is at present no regular pattern on the saint's feast day but the well may be visited at any time by people seeking cures. There are no set prayers but people say their own prayers and drink some of the water. If the pilgrim is seeking a cure, it is necessary to make three separate visits. People in the neighbourhood have no doubts about the cures which have been obtained by visiting the well and among other things I was assured that cases of cancer had been cured.

There is a well dedicated to Saint Brigid in the parish of Outeragh in County Leitrim. It is visited by large numbers of people on the saint's feast day, the 1st of February, but may also be visited on a number of Saturdays during the year. The ritual consists of the rosary as the pilgrim approaches the old graveyard. It is then necessary to say three Hail Marys as he walks around three ancient trees. Formerly the

pilgrims used to kneel at a stone on which a human face had
been carved which was supposed to represent Saint Brigid,
but when the stone was cleaned it was seen to be a corbel
and the face had a beard. Some small sums of money were
sometimes left near the stone and occasionally eggs were left.
When this was done, it was necessary to go to Saint Brigid's
Well about half a mile away, where more prayers were said.
The pilgrim then walked around the well three times, drank
some of the water and said some more prayers.

Some people do this pilgrimage seeking cures for toothache and sore throat and it has the unusual quality that it
may be done on behalf of the sufferer by one of his friends.
This pilgrimage may well be pre-Christian in origin. The
eggs, i.e. the first fruits of the new year, may be part of the
offerings to the god on the first day of the Irish spring. The
walking around the trees also looks like part of a pagan survival.

There is another well dedicated to Saint Brigid about
half a mile from the village of Ardagh in County Longford.
It is also visited on the 1st of February and on a number of
other days, but the visit may be made on any day by people
seeking cures. There are no set prayers or other ritual, but
people pray and drink the well water. When I enquired
about the well and its healing powers, I was told that it has
been known to cure many diseases. The usual cures are skin
rashes, in addition to warts and sore eyes, but its peculiar
quality is to cure people who are 'delicate'.

Not all the wells are very old. On the edge of the
Curragh and a little more than two miles from Kildare
town there is a well at which many cures are said to have
taken place. Two plaques give the essential facts. One reads:

The Blessed Well of Fr. Moore.
Father John Moore was born in 1779 and resided here.
He was ordained in Maynooth in 1803 and was curate
in the parish of Allen. He died on the 12th of March
1826 aged 47 years. He was buried at Allen.

Father Moore's wonderful power is shown by the many
cures and favours obtained by those who carry out the
stations and traditional prayer at the well.

The second plaque reads:

Fr. Moore's Well
Traditional Prayers

1st The Rosary of the Blessed Virgin Mary.
2nd Cross the stepping stones from north to south. Pray for Father Moore, for his parents and for your own intention bathing the affected ailment (if any) with the water.
3rd Three Hail Marys in honour of the Purification of the Blessed Virgin Mary. One visit is then complete.

Three visits should be made for your intention. They are usually done on Fridays and Sundays and should include Confession and Holy Communion.

There is a shrine with a statue of Our Lady, surrounded by the usual votive offerings, an old crutch, medals, rosary beads and holy pictures. Most striking of all was a baby's soother left there no doubt by a grateful mother who believed that her baby had been cured by visiting the well.

The well itself, a spring, is in a circular basin about six feet in diameter with an area of concrete around it and surrounded by a wall. Two stepping stones in the water are those referred to on the plaque.

While I was at the well—on a Friday—two other cars came bringing pilgrims and I was told that thirty cars can be seen at the well on a Sunday in summer. I could not learn of any cure that had been scientifically verified, but many people were prepared to tell me about people who had been cured.

There is another modern well near Ballygar in County Galway. It is in the townland of Tully and on the farm of Mr. Tim Ward. It appears that about the year 1840 a man named Kelly had a daughter who was born blind. This man dreamed that she should go to the well and bathe her eyes in the water. She did this and was cured. Ever since people who suffered from eye diseases visit the well and bathe their eyes in the water. Everyone in the neighbourhood agrees that some people are cured at the well.

A third modern well is at Kilmihil in County Clare. The

traditional story of its origin is that a girl called O'Gorman living in the townland of Tullach Ryan about two hundred years ago suffered from some form of paralysis. On three successive nights she dreamed that if she went to a certain spot and pulled up a pollóg (clump) of rushes water would gush up at the spot. She went and pulled up the rushes and when the water gushed up she drank it and her paralysis was cured.

Since then the well has been visited by the local people and many claim to have been cured by drinking the water, saying the prescribed prayers and doing the official station rounds. I heard of an epileptic child who was believed to have been cured there. The child was taken to the well and given the water to drink. During the night following the visit the patient had a very severe seizure but he never had another one. A patient suffering from advanced bone tuber- culosis was also said to have been cured.

About forty years ago a curate of the parish, Father O'Reilly, organised the people and with the help of a friend, an architect, built an elaborate shrine around the well. The season for making the station is from the 7th of May until the 7th of October, and with an open air Mass on the feast of Saint Michael. The round of the station is made barefoot and would take at least two hours to complete. Whatever the explanation may be, there is little doubt that people have been cured at this holy well.

I do not know if the healing power of any of these wells has been investigated using the standards of the medicine of the second half of the twentieth century. It is unlikely that any of them have been so investigated and this is not very important because it is impossible to assess the value of people's faith. It is certain that many intelligent people are satisfied that some cases of illness are cured by doing stations at these wells. There is not much evidence that people will cease to visit these places. The popularity of some of them may decline and probably there are fewer rags tied on bushes than there were a hundred years ago, but the popularity of others appears to be increasing. Many people feel better and happier for doing these stations and it would be a loss to everybody if a narrow, ignorant materialism caused people to lose faith in them.

CHAPTER II

Spa Wells

It is a little difficult to define what is meant by a spa well.
In a general way, a spa well may be defined as a well, the
waters of which contain salts which are not present in significant amounts in ordinary potable water. I do not know if the
native Irish paid any attention to these strange waters, but it
seems most unlikely that they did; I do not know of any
references to them earlier than the seventeenth century. This
was the time when official medicine became interested in
them and spas on the Continent and in England became
famous and fashionable. Some of them, Bath and Buxton
for example, had been used by the Romans, but the great
popularity of this form of treatment extended from early in
the seventeenth century until the end of the nineteenth century. At present the waters of Bath, Buxton and Harrogate
attract many people and in Ireland the waters of Lisdoon-
varna are still famous. Even yet, bottles of the waters of
famous Continental spas with exotic labels can be found in
some old-fashioned chemist shops, but they are no longer
used to any extent.

The sites of spa wells are marked on the Ordnance Survey
maps and the wells are mentioned in the name books. They
are classified as chalybeate, when the water contains iron
salts, and sulphureous, in which the sulphates are the most
usual salts. The custom was to drink large quantities of the
waters—as much as two gallons a day—and while drinking
it many people agreed that they felt better. The chalybeate
waters, if drunk in large quantities, would probably help to

correct an iron deficiency anaemia. For anyone suffering from chronic constipation—and the wealthy often did during the seventeenth and eighteenth centuries—waters containing sulphates would be helpful. Epsom salts (magnesium sulphate) and Glauber's salts (sodium sulphate) are examples of these. Perhaps the large volume of water drunk was as important as anything else. The water is excreted through the kidneys and it might well help to wash out small pieces of gravel and it would also help in cases of infection of the kidney.

There have been a number of books written on the Irish spa wells during the days of their fame. An early reference to Irish spas is a letter to the Duke of Ormond by Doctor Edmund O'Meara in 1674. The doctor advised the Duke, his patient, to drink spa water, leaving it to the Duke himself to decide which spa here or in England he would prefer. A small book called 'The Irish Spaw' by Doctor Peter Bellon was published in Dublin in 1684. There was a number of other books written during the eighteenth century and probably the best of these was 'The Mineral Waters of Ireland' by John Rutty, published in Dublin in 1757.

It will be noticed that in the course of this book forge water has been mentioned as a treatment for tiredness and some other conditions. In describing the spa wells, Rutty said that some of them smelled like forge water. This may have been the source of the belief in the usefulness of forge water, which was probably rich in salts of iron and if taken continuously would help a case of anaemia due to iron deficiency.

Using Rutty's book as a guide, I visited a number of the wells and enquired on the spot about the use of the waters at present. Rutty made mention of a number of wells containing purging waters which were in use in the city of Dublin. These were in the neighbourhood of Francis Street, the Coombe and Thomas Court, and he mentions five of these wells in Francis Street. These were at the Burn's Arms, the Pump, the Plough, Vernon's Head and the Wheat Sheaf. These wells are now almost completely forgotten, but one man was able to tell me about Parkes' Joiner's shop opposite the old Weavers' Hall in the Coombe, where there was a well where people were welcome to drink the spa water. It was

said to help cases of rheumatism and was used to cure hang-
overs. Rutty mentioned other wells in the neighbourhood at
Ballydowd, Howth, St. Margaret's, and Templeogue, but
these are no longer used and even the Lucan well, which was
so long famous, is now used much less than formerly.

I visited the spa well at Swanlinbar in County Cavan
during the present summer (1971). It had not changed since I
went there over twenty years ago to get some water for my
mother, who said it made her much better. It still had the
smell of rotten eggs, perceptible from several yards, and the
path to the well from the road was still used. This well was
very famous during the eighteenth century and Rutty de-
voted more than forty pages of his book to its wonderful
powers to cure almost every disease, even including a case or
two of leprosy. When people walked to Lough Derg on pilgrimage, the custom was to stop at the well and drink the
water before proceeding on the journey.

Rutty also mentioned a number of spa wells in the neighbourhood of Drumsna in County Leitrim. I went there
recently and found that two of them are still known; one is
at MacManus's Cross on the road between Jamestown and
Carrick-on-Shannon. The water of this well is still used to
cure worms in children and in horses. The other is on the
land owned by Mr. Bernard Garvey, near Drumsna. It is
little used, but is believed to cure worms and is also good
for aches and pains. I was interested to hear that the people
of Drumsna do not want to talk about spa water, except to
complain about it. All the local water is spa water and they
cannot get a suitable supply of fresh water for the little town.

Around Slieve an Iarainn in County Leitrim there are
many spa wells; I examined the maps of the district in the
Ordnance Office and found at least twenty such wells entered
on the maps. People still know where they are, but few
people now drink the waters. This decline in their use may
be due to the fall in the population of the mountainous district of County Leitrim.

It would seem that the use of spa water is now no longer
used in folk medicine, but as an illustration of its importance I will end with a quotation from Rutty's book about
the chalybeate waters of a well near Wexford. This is from

a letter written to Rutty by Peter Sweetman, Physician at Wexford:

> It would be endless to enumerate all the disorders in which these salutary waters are drank: the chlorosis, obstructed and immoderate menstrua, bilious and nervous colicks, the Gohorrhoea Simplex, Fluor Albus, Barrenness, Jaundice, cachexy, the Hypochondriac disease, Gravel, loss of appetite and scurvy, are diseases mostly relieved and often cured by the long protracted use of these waters.

CHAPTER III

Sweat-houses

IN certain parts of County Leitrim disused sweat-houses can still be seen—an average of one per townland in some areas. My grandmother, who came from Tullywan high on the side of Slieve an Iarainn, told me she had often used the townland sweat-house and felt very much better and cleaner for it. An old man, my granduncle, who had suffered with rheumatism for many years, also told me that he had used it and said that a good sweat gave him considerable relief from his aches and pains. That was its great use, the relief of aches and pains in men, while women used is as a way of bathing and as a beauty treatment. On the 6″ maps of the district the sites of the sweat-houses were shown, and for a long time I assumed that these sites could be found in almost every part of Ireland. If they were ever so widespread is doubtful and in most parts of the country their use has been completely forgotten.

There has been a number of references to them in the Journal of the Royal Society of Antiquaries of Ireland and in the Ulster Journal of Archaeology. In the Ulster Journal there have been recent articles on the sweat-houses of Counties Derry, Cavan, Tyrone and Fermanagh. In the Journal of the Royal Society of Antiquaries sweat-houses on Rathlin Island, County Donegal (near Ballyshannon), County Sligo (Inishmurry) and County Tyrone have been mentioned. There is also mention of the remains of a number of sweat-houses in County Louth. In County Leitrim I was able to identify the remains of forty-six in the district around Lough Allen and Slieve an Iarainn. Outside these areas, in the drumlin country of County Leitrim, there were neither remains of them nor traditions of their use and their use has also been forgotten in the east of County Cavan.

I recently visited a very well preserved one in County Galway. It can be found about a mile from Barnderg on the left hand side of the road to Tuam. It is approached by a stile and is about fifty yards from the road. The house is very well built, about ten feet square, five feet high and with a stone roof. The doorway is about two feet six inches by two feet. Beside it is a well surrounded by a well-built wall and with steps down to the water. The ground around it is rather soft, but otherwise two men could get it ready for use in about half a day by cutting a few bushes and spreading some sand on the soft ground. This is the only example of a square-built sweat-house which I have found.

Outside the province of Ulster and the adjacent counties they are quite unknown. I have been unable to find any traditions of them in Counties Mayo, Clare or Kerry.

All the descriptions of them agree closely. They are circular or oval, built of stones and clay and often with a roof of flagstones with a hole somewhere in the roof to act as a vent for the smoke. In some cases the floor was covered with flagstones or cobbles, but generally it was beaten clay. On the average, the place was about five feet in diameter, but some of those described in County Londonderry were oval, about seven feet long, three feet wide and five feet high. Many, but not all, were built near a stream or a well. The door was always small; it was necessary to crawl inside.

The procedure was to light a large turf fire inside the house and keep it burning for a number of days so that the house would be thoroughly warmed up. When this was done the bather crept in, taking green rushes to protect his feet and a bundle of them on which to sit while he sweated in the heat. There might also be squares of scraw (the top of the bog) used to protect the feet. In some cases water was sprinkled on the flagstones or cobbles to make a steam bath. The doorway was stuffed with the bather's clothing or in some other way to conserve the heat.

It was usual to use the hot bath during the summer or autumn; in County Leitrim, where many of the sweat-houses are above the thousand feet contour line, the winter is cold and wet. Also it was not usual to bathe alone and, as an additional precaution, someone waited outside in case one of the bathers got weak and had to be taken out. When the bather was finished, he came out and had a cold plunge in the nearby stream and then wrapped up warmly and went home to bed.

In the name books of the 25″ maps of County Leitrim, the sweat-houses are mentioned and in some cases a short description is given. In Sheet No. 18 there is a description of one at Derrinvoher:

> (The name) applies to a small rude structure built of stones and clay and resembling a beehive in shape. It is used for the cure of certain diseases, principally rheumatism, by means of artificial heat to induce excessive perspiration. The building is heated inside by peat fires which are then removed and the patient goes in by a small opening or doorway, and remains until the cure is supposed to have taken effect.

Haliday Sutherland in his book 'Lapland Journey' describes the Finnish sauna bath, now a popular form of treatment for something or other. Perhaps a modern style sweat-house, called a Teach Alluis of course, might become popular if it were installed in some of our more expensive hotels. It might even become one of the attractions of this country.

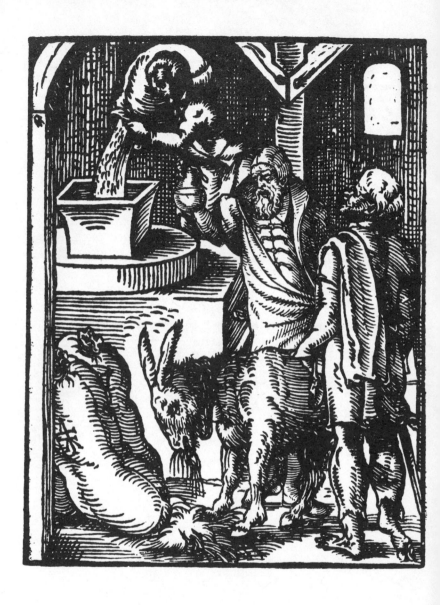

Part 4

Veterinary Medicine

CHAPTER I

Diseases of Horses

INTRODUCTION

Veterinary folk medicine is almost forgotten. In order to learn about the treatments used it is necessary to ask elderly men who could have used the treatments; few young men, unless they had seen their fathers use them, know anything about them. Today, if a farmer has a sick cow he is certain to consult a veterinary surgeon and will do exactly as he is advised. Many farmers nowadays read farming journals and Department of Agriculture leaflets about the care of domestic animals. In making up animal foods, all modern knowledge of dietetics is used. This is very necessary in preparing foods for animals who have no natural source of food—battery fed chickens, for example—because unless the feed provides all the necessary ingredients the animals will suffer from deficiency diseases. Most domestic animals are now inoculated against the usual infectious diseases so that the loss from these diseases is now very low. All this is recognised as good animal husbandry and if at present a farmer were to use a folk remedy to treat one of his stock it would be a matter for comment among his neighbours. Few would think it strange if he were to take yellow flowers to cure his jaundice, or gave what a ferret had not eaten to his child to cure whooping cough.

Recently I heard a story of a folk veterinary surgeon, now dead, who lived in County Meath. He used mainly herbal remedies and it was necessary that some of the herbs be gathered before sunrise and it was also necessary that while out gathering them he must not meet anyone. One morning, to his annoyance, as he was returning home he met one of his neighbours. 'Bad luck to you,' he said, 'you set me back nine days.'

DISEASES OF HORSES

There are two short tracts on diseases of horses written in the Irish language. One of these was written in the sixteenth century, and the other may be somewhat older. Both have been edited and translated by Professor Brian Ó Cuiv and were published in Celtica Volume II. Some of the treatments advised in these tracts have continued in use as folk remedies and reference will be made to these in the course of this chapter.

In the records of the Leinster Irish army during the Confederate Wars there is a reference dated 26th May 1646. This is an order to pay 18/2 to John Bellew for Thomas Tylin 'Smith and farrier', being a week's pay to 1 June and 10/- to buy drugs. This is the earliest reference I know to an official veterinary surgeon in an Irish army, but no doubt there were always men who took care of the horses and until very recently the smith was the local horse doctor. My friend Mr. Thomas Cosgrove of Ballinamore is my great source of information about the treatment of horses.

VETERINARY MALPRAXIS

There were a number of methods used to disguise faults in a horse, all of which show a high degree of ingenuity. In some cases the back muscles may be less well developed on one side than on the other. This may be disguised by putting a strong plaster of mustard or belladonna over the weaker muscles. The irritation by the plaster will cause a swelling and disguise the weak muscles. A more crude method is to prod the area with a cobbler's awl, in the hope of causing the necessary swelling. I was told that this method should only be used by an expert because the exact degree of swelling must be judged carefully.

If a horse is going slightly lame an old trick is to get a man with very bad feet to lead him. The slight lameness is not then so likely to be noticed.

A vicious horse may be made quiet for a short time by giving this sedative mixture:

Chloral Hydrate   1 ounce
Potassium Bromide   1 ounce
Sweeten with sugar.
All is given in one dose in a pint of water.

An older method is to give the horse parsley—as much as he can be persuaded to eat.

There is a simple trick to deceive a buyer about a broken winded horse. The person showing the horse puts on a curb bit to ride him past the inspecting veterinary surgeon. As the rider passes, he drops his hands, relaxes the curb chain and the horse will breathe easily for a moment or so. It is difficult to believe that this trick could deceive anyone, but I have been assured that it has done so.

The ritual of making an old broken-down horse look young is quite an elaborate one. If the horse is going lame, he is fired and the mark of the iron disguised with a piece of dirt, or better still with a dressing of train-oil. The teeth require expert attention. A blacksmith's rasp is used to file the inside of the upper teeth and the outside of the lower teeth, and as an additional refinement the proper marks are made on the teeth with a hot iron. Next the grey hairs around the horse's mouth are dyed with a hair dye. The most skilful part of the work is on the eyes. A hypodermic needle attached to a bicycle pump is inserted into the outer corner of the eye, through the conjunctiva, and air is blown in behind the eye to fill out the eye socket. Last, when the animal has defecated, a piece of ginger previously well chewed is placed in the rectum of the horse. This causes pain and makes the animal restless.

Once in my life, at about the age of ten, on a fair morning I had a chance to see all this carried out. Normally children would be chased away, but I must have looked harmlessly dimwitted. It took a lot of careful questioning in later years to learn exactly how the filing of the teeth was done, as well as all the other details, but I have been assured by experts that my details are correct.

COLIC
This is a vague diagnosis. It means that the horse is uncomfortable, is not eating and has a swollen belly. As these

signs may be due to a number of causes, there are two
methods of treatment, one of which seems to be the opposite
of the other. One method was to keep the horse moving and
if necessary put on a saddle and ride him. This was done to
prevent the horse from lying down or rolling over, because if
he did it was feared that he might twist a gut. The other
method was to bed the stall well with clean straw. The horse
was then given a dose of laudanum—'about an ounce'—and
as the laudanum took effect the horse was likely to lie down
and go to sleep. It was hoped that when the effect of the
laudanum had worn off the colic would be relieved.

Either method would work if the colic was due to an over-
loaded gut, but in the rare case of a twisted gut the animal
would almost certainly die no matter what treatment was
given.

BROKEN WIND

In this condition a horse, when he is worked, experiences
difficulty in breathing due to spasm of the larynx. One
method of treatment was to give the horse the white of a
dozen eggs every morning for a week.

In other cases, a tin of archangel tar—about a pound—
was placed at the bottom of a barrel of water from which the
horse drank. After a few days a slight scum will be seen on
the top of the water and the horse will probably refuse to
drink. He must then be kept without water until he does
drink the water, and after a few days he may continue to
drink it without protest. This treatment must be continued
for a long time.

Tar water has a notable history. During the eighteenth
century George Berkeley, the famous Bishop of Cloyne, advo-
cated the use of tar water as a treatment for many diseases
and a famous pamphlet which he wrote on the subject made
its use popular. This is the only use of tar water in folk
medicine of which I have heard.

WORMS AND BOTTS

One treatment advised for worms was the tops of furze
bushes. The tops were cut with a reaping hook (sickle) and
pounded on a block with a mallet. The furze was then given

to the horse. I have been told that this treatment is very successful, especially if given with a pint of linseed oil. K'eogh says that the seed of furze is good to kill worms.

Another method of treating worms appears to have been taken over from official medicine. The preparation contained:

Croton seeds	35 grains
Aniseeds	20 grains
Linseed	1 dram
Bolus Armenicus	Enough to make up the dose.

This is given to the horse in a sloppy mash and he is kept in the stable for twenty-four hours. He is then ridden and it is expected that he will pass the worms.

The botts is a common condition in horses. It is believed to be caused by the horse licking his legs where a fly had laid eggs; in that way the infection reaches the stomach of the horse where the eggs hatch out. The treatment is to give the horse a gallon of milk well sweetened with sugar. When this has been done, the horse is thrown and turned on his back. The botts loose their grip on the lining of the stomach to drink the milk and are passed out.

In some parts of County Clare botts and worms are treated by having the horse drink the water of Moy-Lacha lake. The lake is near Kilrush and the power of the water is attributed to Saint Sennan, the local saint.

An official preparation which became a folk treatment in County Longford contained:

Carbon Disulphide	5 drams
Turpentine	2 drams
Linseed oil	10 ounces

This mixture is given in the morning and two hours afterwards a further pint of linseed oil is given.

FARCEY

This is essentially an incurable condition in which one of the hind legs of the horse becomes greatly swollen due to venous thrombosis. In County Wicklow it has been treated by the touch of a seventh son and some prayers. On the

Meath-Cavan border the bog mud of a dried-up lake, Lough Leighis, was applied as a large poultice to the swollen leg.

In County Leitrim a more active form of treatment was used. The horse was first bled from the swollen leg and about a quart of blood removed. He was then fasted for twenty-four hours and at the end of that time he was given a physic containing a pint of linseed oil and a glass of turpentine. This will make the animal sick. He must then be taken out and ridden until he defecates. The swollen leg is then bandaged smoothly and firmly—'like a puttee'—from below upwards. The bandage is renewed as necessary and the horse must be left on grass for about six weeks.

GREASY HEELS

This condition of the hooves is caused by leaving the manure under the horse's feet in the stall. It is first necessary to clean out the stall properly and keep it clean. The feet are then thoroughly washed with strong black carbolic soap and the washing is repeated daily for a week. This would probably clear up a mild case. If it is slow to clear up, the feet may be dressed twice with archangel tar.

In more severe cases, in addition to the ordinary cleaning, one may use the size of a thumb of bluestone dissolved in water to dress the heels. There is a number of poultices which may be used. One may be made of grated raw carrots which is applied daily for three days. It is then advised to change to a bread poultice. The bread is soaked in water and the hard crusts removed. The soft bread is spread on a cloth and covered with cream and applied to the feet.

If all these methods fail, a poultice of human dung is certain to succeed. In order to make it less offensive, flour is added and the mixture made up with a trowel. It may be necessary to repeat the dressing a few times, but it is the best method of treating greasy heels. K'eogh is an advocate of the use of poultices of human dung for many conditions. This is what he wrote:

> The ordure or dung outwardly applied is good against scald heads, gouts, cancers, strumaes, inflammations in wounds, mortifications, an ulcerated erysipelas, and the quinsy.

He has more to say about the virtues of human dung, but that will do. With such wonderful powers it would be expected to cure a simple condition like greasy heels without delay.

Thrush in the frog may be treated by cleaning out the crack as completely as possible and then filling it with roasted salt. A plug of wadding is then used to keep the salt in position.

SKIN DISEASES

Warts: The usual method was to cut the warts off with a sharp-edged pincers and cauterise the raw surface. In the Irish tract on diseases of horses, the method advised is to squeeze the warts with a tongs, but if there were many warts the hot iron was advised.

Scruff: This appears to have been a fungus infection of the skin. It was treated with a mixture of train-oil and sulphur with success. An ointment of equal parts of white lead and zinc ointment was also used to treat scruff.

Itch: This occurs on the hooves of horses and is treated with a saturated solution of bluestone (copper sulphate). The Irish tract gives an elaborate prescription for the treatment of mange in horses. It recommends an:

> ointment of alum, roots of dock (prema copóg) and pepperwort (glaistena) and horse clover (semur capaill) and honey suckle leaves (duille feithe) well crushed and boiled with butter or lard, or both, and strained through a linen cloth, and put salt or sulphur in it. Apply that frequently and it will be healed.

Bashed Knees: Horses going downhill too fast may fall and cut the skin over the knees. If there is any considerable amount of scarring, hair will not grow on the scars and this is considered a notable blemish. The scars may be disguised by applying a mixture of train-oil and sulphur. Another method is to cover the scars with the ashes of burned bark or the ashes may be added to the train oil and sulphur. The reason for this elaborate form of disguise appears to be the belief that if a horse has fallen once he is likely to do so again and if the skin of the knees is badly scarred it is assumed that the horse has fallen on a number of occasions.

In sixteenth century Ireland, injured knees in horses appear to have been common and severe. The tracts advise that the injured area be burned with a hot iron if there is thick suppuration like the white of egg. A plaster of sheep's dung, salted butter and the yolk of hen eggs is applied for two or three days. Then well boiled mallow, stalks of dock leaves, and chickweed are all crushed and applied as a plaster with sheep fat and butter.

A similar plaster of elm (bark) well crushed and boiled and made up with sheep fat is also advised as a dressing for injured knees.

Harness Galls: These are best prevented by care in saddling or harnessing the horse. Before harnessing, the pressure areas should be treated with salt and water and then with methylated spirits. If a driver suspects that a gall is forming during a journey, he may treat the area with urine and then with whiskey.

In the Irish tract it is advised that proud flesh be cut off and a dressing of yolk of egg and salt be applied and left until it falls off. The galls are then washed in fresh urine daily for three or four days. Then white of egg and hardened (?) powder are applied. The tract says that alum is also good for harness galls and Irish folk medicine continues this practice by using a mixture of alum and sugar of lead for harness galls. An old preparation for harness galls was a paste made of Fuller's earth and tar, which I was assured would cure the gall very quickly.

DISEASES OF THE FEET

The saying that 'a horse is worth four times the price of his worst foot', expresses the importance of the feet. Due to the complex evolutionary history of the foot of the horse, as well as his walking on hard roads, there are many conditions which occur in the feet of horses and some of these may render him useless.

Hard Feet: This is diagnosed by trying to crack a match on the frog. Normally the frog should be damp and the match will not light. The treatment consisted of a dressing of soft cow dung and, as an alternative, a dressing of linseed oil.

Hot Tendons in the Foot: This condition was treated with a poultice of yellow clay. People who treated diseases of horses kept a supply of suitable clay which in some cases had to be brought from a distance. All the stones were removed and the clay made into a soft mud and applied to the tender area. It was necessary that water be poured over the dressing from time to time to keep the clay soft and wet.

Bony Overgrowths: These are many and include side bones, ring bones, tuiret pins and curbs. These are all treated by blistering. There were two blistering preparations used, each containing much the same ingredients. One was:

Red Iodide of Mercury	2 ounces and 2 drams
White Wax	7 drams
Oil of Nux Vomica	$4\frac{1}{2}$ ounces
Pure Lard	6 ounces and 2 drams
Cantharides Powder	$1\frac{1}{2}$ ounces

When this has been made up it is believed to become stronger if kept for a week.

The hair is clipped off the area to be blistered and the blistering preparation rubbed in for fifteen minutes with the little finger side of the hand—the palm or the fingers should not be used. A smoothing iron, heated, is held over the area 'to drive the blisters inwards'. When all this has been done, the horse must be tied up to prevent him from biting the blistered area. After three days get a pint of sweet oil and allow the oil to seep down slowly through the hair and on to the treated area. This treatment with the sweet oil is continued every day for a week. I have been assured that if this treatment is carried out properly a side bone will be eaten away.

Sand Cracks in the Hooves: The same blistering procedure is used as in the treatment of side bone. In this case it is most important that the sides of the hoof and the front be not blistered at the same time. If the entire hoof is treated at the same time, the blister may kill the growth of the hoof. My informant told me that as a young apprentice he had seen the hoof killed in this way and the horse made useless.

A less severe blister may be prepared with melted goose-grease to which turpentine and the juice of turpeen (house leek) has been added.

Bone Overgrown in the Foot: This condition may be disguised, but it requires an expert horse coper to do it. The method is to strike the horse a blow on the opposite foot in the exact spot where the overgrowth is. Expertly done, this will cause a swelling corresponding to the overgrowth and both may pass as normal.

LAMPERS

This condition presents as an unpleasant looking crop of blisters which form inside the mouth and is usually associated with bad teeth. The old treatment was to cut the tops of furze bushes, break them up very fine and mix them with the horse's mash. When the horse eats the furze the thorns stick in the blisters and he licks them to get the thorns out. In this way it is hoped to cure the condition. A more radical method is to operate on and open the blisters. The blade of a small knife is passed through a cork until no more than a quarter of an inch is outside. Two big scars are made from side to side through the blistered area and three or four from front to back, but the operator must be careful not to go too deeply, as he may cause severe bleeding. The scars are then rubbed with a fistful of salt. The horse will then lick and suck the blisters as he was expected to do when the thorns stuck in them. Still another method, if the operator is afraid of bleeding, is to burn the blistered area with a hot iron and rub in salt as usual.

BLEEDING

If for any reason a horse is bleeding, it is the common practice to feed him on green cabbage. As a local dressing, a fungus called 'the buck mushroom' (an pocán) is used. The usual name in English is 'puff-ball' and it is the yellow dust—the spores—which is sprinkled on the bleeding area. These spores are also used to stop bleeding in human beings.

DIABETES IN HORSES

This is a condition which is most usually seen in yearlings.

The usual method is to put bread soda in the drinking water. A more elaborate preparation contained:

Potassium Iodide	3	ounces
Sodium Iodide	3	ounces
Iron Sulphate	4	ounces
Water, to	20	ounces

One ounce of the mixture was given three times a day.

INJURED SHOULDER

This injury is quite common in horses and it used be treated with what was called a soap blister. Soap and water were massaged on the skin and the muscles around the tender area. The massage was carried out twice a day and the treatment was continued as long as necessary. Similarly, the soap blister and massage were used for sprains and muscle injuries generally and were often of great benefit. In the sixteenth century a horse with a sprain was treated with a plaster of dock leaves boiled in water and strained. Unsalted butter was then added to the boiled leaves to make up the plaster.

COUGH

This does not appear to have been regarded as a very serious condition. It was usually cleared up fairly quickly with a mustard blister applied to the lower jaw and around the jowls. A similar condition, strangles, was treated with warm salt.

The mediaeval Irish veterinary surgeon was very familiar with strangles. He treated the condition with primrose roots crushed well and strained into breast milk or whey of goat's milk, and the directions were:

Put them in the nose frequently according to your discretion.

DIET

Bleed him and physic him and put him out to grass.
This expression sums up the treatment of a horse who had been overworked and badly cared for. Bleeding was routine practice in human medicine until comparatively recent times,

so it could not be expected that horses would escape. Probably it did less harm to the horses because it was not as easy
to get blood out of a horse as out of a human patient. Physic
in this case meant a pound of Epsom salts and an ounce of
nitre dissolved in water. This would act as a strong purgative
and would not do any good, but could not do any harm
either. The putting out to grass was the important thing. The
shoes would be taken off and on the soft grass his feet would
improve. The rest would improve him considerably and feeding on good fresh grass—the natural food of the horse—would
improve his general health. It is likely that, due to constant
feeding on hay and oats, he would suffer from some dietetic
deficiency diseases and these would be corrected by the grass.

It was usual to treat city working horses in this way. Every
year when the grass was fresh they were sent off to the
country to graze on the grass. In these cases the hard streets
would damage their feet and the month out on grass without
shoes would be of great benefit.

SHOEING

Skilful shoeing can correct certain defects of the action.
Probably the most common of these is called brushing. In
this case as the horse brings one hind foot past the other he
strikes the opposite foot. This could be a disabling defect,
but most cases can be corrected by a skilful farrier. In dressing
the hoof, he takes care to see that the outside of the hoof is
lower than the inside. To increase this further, the shoe is
made higher on the inside and tapered carefully from the
toe.

PSYCHOLOGICAL DISORDERS

There are a number of conditions, more usually found in
racehorses in training, which would be classified as neurosis
if they were found occurring in human patients. When a
horse is in training he is alone in a loose box with no contact with other horses and this must cause trouble in an
animal who would run naturally with a herd. One of these
conditions is what horsey people call 'crib biting'. The crib
biter uses his teeth on the wooden horizontal bar on the
top of his manger. He will even bite on a metal top. I have

not heard of any form of treatment other than to ensure that there is no horizontal bar within his reach.

In other cases the horse is described as 'a stall walker', and again this does not occur when horses are running together. The horse walks round and round in his stall and efforts have been made to stop him by putting bales of hay and such things in his way. None of these measures make any difference. The condition is probably due to loneliness and will stop if he is let run with other horses. If a goat is put in the box with him it may help, but a better method is to break a large hole in one of the walls so that he can see the horse in the next box. As it almost always occurs in horses in training, the natural treatment is rather difficult.

Sometimes a horse refuses to eat. Here the method used is the same as one used to persuade a child to eat. A hole is made in the wall and a greedy horse is put in the next stall. Things are so arranged that the greedy horse can see and nearly reach the neglected food in the other stall. He will make every effort to reach it and if he does succeed in eating some of it the first horse will probably eat it rather than leave it to the greedy fellow.

Dung eating may also be a neurosis. It is treated by mixing egg shells with dung, hoping that the shells will hurt the inside of his mouth. A more drastic method is to mix red pepper with the dung.

CHAPTER II

Diseases of Cattle

Go mbéidh cach bó agat go deoidh.

THIS Irish expression, which was said to the woman of the house when she gave someone a drink of milk, may be translated:

May you always have cow dung.

It indicates the importance of the cow in the economy of the country and in the social life of the community. In the native Irish annals epizootics are mentioned many times and a severe one could be as great a disaster as an epidemic. A very unpleasant feature of Irish wars up to the end of the seventeenth century was the famine which followed the driving off of the cattle; this was the method used by the English in winning wars in Ireland. I will only quote one such reference to an epizootic which occurred about the years 1321-1326:

1321 Great cow distruction (bodith) throughout all Ireland (Annals of Lough Ce).

1324 Cow disease called the Mael Domhnaigh (Annals of Louth Ce).

1325 Some cow distruction (Annals of Ulster).

1326 Great disease on cows. Great famine (Annals of Innisfallen).

There were certain measures necessary to protect the cow. When a heifer had her first calf it was necessary that any excess hair around the udder must be burned off with the flame of a blessed candle which was passed from before backwards and between the hind legs of the animal. This ritual was carried out to ensure a good yield of milk.

Every time a cow calved, there was a ritual performed which might be compared to churching after the birth of a child. A lighted candle was passed from one side of the cow across the back, under the belly and backwards between the legs. I was not able to learn what prayers were said during either of these ceremonies, but probably there were some.

When a cow had been milked, the milker must put a finger in the milk and make the Sign of the Cross with the milk on the flank of the cow and say: 'God bless the cow'. If someone entered the byre and did not say 'God bless the cows', this would be disapproved of, and if he were a Catholic he might be suspect. Protestants were excused this duty. It would be bad mannered if one were given a drink of milk and did not say it.

Another method of protecting the cows was to hang up a Saint Brigid's cross in the byre. The legends about Saint Brigid often mention the fact that she protected cattle. At Saint Brigid's Well in my native parish she is reputed to have restored to life the only cow of a widow. The story said that the cow had been killed by dogs. In statues of the saint she is sometimes shown with a cow in her arms. The tradition may be very old because Brigit was the name of the Irish goddess of healing.

It was believed in County Leitrim that certain people had the evil eye. The belief was vague and it was difficult to get people to speak openly about it, but I remember one man who believed that one of his neighbours had the evil eye and on no account would he let him into his byre to look at the cows. The fact that the neighbour was rather self-important, not very well liked, and a Protestant to boot, may have had something to do with the belief and perhaps in some other parts of Ireland some Catholic might be believed to have the evil eye for equally logical reasons. I have also heard of a way to injure one's neighbour's cattle. The person who wishes to do this makes a model in wax of the person whose cattle he wishes to injure. Pins are stuck in the wax, which is then thrown across the fence into the neighbour's field. If this were done it was believed that the cows in the field would die.

Another danger was what was called the gae sidhe (fairy

dart). Stone Age arrowheads are sometimes found in Ireland.
These were believed to have been shot by fairies and might
injure people, but more usually they were shot at cattle.
If an animal was not thriving, people used wonder if it had
been elf shot and a folk curer was usually called in for con-
sultation. His method was to examine the animal to try to
find where the fairy dart had struck it. He then measured the
animal three times round the belly, and that completed the
cure. In other cases the curer gave the animal water to drink.
One of the arrowheads was placed in the water. Wood-
Martin gives many details of this cure.

The most usual method of protecting cattle against bad
fairies and the evil eye is to tie a piece of red cloth around
the animal's tail. This is also a very old custom. Red is the
colour used to resist and expel demons and ward off other
evil influences.

The fear of taking butter was universal. It was believed
that some people could steal their neighbour's butter and
many methods were used to prevent this. If while the churning was being done a visitor called, it was necessary that the
visitor take a turn with the dash. This was to ensure that he
would not take the butter with him when he departed. Anyone who has ever churned with a dash will realise what a
tiring and dull job it is and the story makes sure that every
visitor will give a hand with the churning. Another method
of protecting the butter was to put a garland woven of twigs
of the boor tree (elderberry) on the lid of the churn. The
garland was called the caolach chaorthainn and it ensured
that the butter would not be taken. The use of the elderberry appears to be modern because the word caorthann
means the rowan tree and was originally used.

VETERINARY MALPRAXIS

There are certain practices of which I have heard which
may be of interest. There is a method of making the tuberculin test negative. Once I was asked how this could be done
and, although I have had some experience of the use of
tuberculin, it took some time to work out the method. If
one wishes to have a negative result, 2cc of tuberculin are
injected under the skin of the belly. In the case of a positive

reaction there will be a very strong reaction, but the swelling will not be noticed. When a week or so later another injection of tuberculin is given, the animal's body will be unable to react to the tuberculin and the test is found to be negative.

If, on the other hand, a positive tuberculin reaction is required, this may also be obtained. When the veterinary surgeon has given his injection, this is followed in the same spot by an injection of about 2cc of turpentine. This will cause a severe local reaction which will probably be read as positive.

One can estimate the number of calves a cow has had by counting the rings on her horns. In order to make her younger, it was not unusual to pare the rings away and then smooth down the horns with a blacksmith's rasp. The job was finished by rubbing the horns with the wax from the animal's ears.

MAJOR SURGERY

The two major surgical procedures in cattle were dehorning and castrating and I have never known an official veterinary surgeon to be required for these. Both procedures are now obsolete. In castrating there were two major problems, to control bleeding and prevent the wounds becoming infected. The control of bleeding is especially important because the blood supply of the testes comes directly from the main blood vessel of the body and unless care was taken to control the bleeding the animal might bleed to death. Similarly the control of infection was important. If the animal were put in a house after the operation, the wound would become severely infected. As an additional precaution, the operation wounds were left open to allow the wound to drain freely.

In performing the operation it was necessary that the animal be tossed and four experienced men were needed. An iron ring about three inches in diameter was tied between the hind legs to the metatarsus of each foot. A loop of rope was then placed around the animal's neck, so tied that it would not become tighter when pulled upon. A long rope from the loop was then taken backwards between the forelegs through the iron ring, back along the left side and through the loop around the animal's neck. In the case of a larger animal—a mature bull for instance—two ropes might be used, one being brought through the loop on either side of the head. By pulling on the rope it was not very difficult to get the animal down and secured safely.

The operator made an incision extending from the middle of the right side of the scrotum to the bottom and took the right testis out of the sac. Care was necessary in freeing the spermatic cord, because there was a danger of injuring the artery. A piece of elderberry stick about six inches long and an inch thick was split evenly down the middle and the soft pith removed. This was replaced with a mixture of oaten meal and archangel tar. In County Leitrim the stick was called a clam and further north a clem, probably a local pronunciation of the word clamp. Grooves had been cut in both ends of the clam and one end was tied with strong cord, using the groove to make sure that it would not slip. The two pieces of stick were then placed around the cord and tied firmly to act as a ligature and stop the flow of blood to the testis. The operation was then done on the opposite side. During the following week or so the testis atrophied, dried up and fell off.

In order to avoid infection, the procedure was carried out in a field and the animals were immediately put out to grass. Everyone was warned about the danger of infection and castration was always carried out in the early summer when grass was plentiful and the weather fine and before there were many flies about.

Dehorning appears to have been a much more painful procedure. No anaesthetic was used and the horn was quickly taken off by a saw which resembled an old-fashioned amputation saw. This was a necessary operation if the bullocks were to be fattened in a stockyard. The wounds were not usually dressed, but if they became heavily infected they were washed with a diluted solution of Jeyes' Fluid.

MILK FEVER

This condition is liable to occur in a very good milking cow who has just calved and begun to produce a large quantity of milk. The condition is due to a low blood calcium because the calcium has been used to form the bones of the calf and has also been put into the milk. When the blood calcium falls below a critical level, the animal collapses. Some mild cases may be helped by giving the cow lime or lime water, but in severe cases the cow may die unless the production of milk can be quickly stopped. This was done by inflating the udder with a bicycle pump. The valve of a bicycle tube is put into each teat in turn and each quadrant inflated. The teats are then tied with wide tapes to keep the air in. This will stop the production of milk and if done with care it will not do grave damage to the udder, and the blood calcium will gradually rise. Clearly this was a method which was taken over from official veterinary practice and could save the life of the cow.

THE BLOAT

This is due to an accumulation of gas in the stomach. It may occur when the animal is first put out in the spring and eats greedily of the fresh grass. The animal is clearly uncomfortable and if the belly is percussed it will give a note like a drum. The condition may be efficiently treated by letting the air out. This used to be done, I have been told, by means of a very thin stiletto-like knife, but I have only seen it done with a long hollow needle which is pushed through the skin and into the bloated area and allows the stomach gas to escape. It is quite an impressive performance and I have never heard of any complications which followed it.

There is a popular mixture which was also used to treat the bloat. It is also a take-over from official medicine and contained:

Ginger	one dram
Wood charcoal	two ounces
Amonium carbonate	one dram
Nux Vomica	half a dram
Sodium hyposulphite	one dram
Gentian	one dram
Baking soda	one dram

This powder is given on thin gruel and repeated in twelve hours. In less severe cases in calves a pint of buttermilk to which three teaspoonsful of soot have been added may be given.

WARTS

It seems strange to find a method which is used for treating warts in children also used for warts in cattle. Saint Monaghan's Well in County Offaly is famous for curing warts in cattle, the warts being bathed in water taken from the well. Some leaves must then be taken from the tree over the well and buried in the ground, and as the leaves decay so will the warts. The significance of this combination of washing and wasting cures has already been discussed.

SORE EYES

For a scum on the cow's eye, the eyes may be bathed in lime water. Another method is to blow calomel into the eye. This appears to be an official remedy which was taken over fairly recently. I cannot say how successful the treatment was, but people said that it worked very well. There was another method which seems to be a true folk cure. This was to hang up an ivy leaf over the fireplace. It will dry and shrivel up and as it does so the sore eye will be getting better.

RED MURRAIN (*Red water*)

This disease is due to a parasite which gets into the red cells of the animal's blood causing the corpuscles to break and releasing the red colouring matter (haemoglobin) into the blood stream. This is passed out in the urine, colouring it red. The object of treatment is to replace the lost blood. The animal is made to eat about a pound of salt. The salt was sometimes mixed with lard. This made it easier to give to the animal. This causes the animal to drink large quantities of water, so washing out the haemoglobin. The animal may also be given gallons of strong tea. This is also a matter of replacing lost fluid. The next cure is a strange one: the animal is given two Reckett's blue tablets. I am unable to suggest any reason for this. Still another treatment was a mixture of mulled porter and treacle.

INFECTED FEET

This may be due to a number of causes, stones between the toes, injury or infection. A stone may be picked out with a big nail or similar sort of instrument. If a light rope can be got in between the toes, sawing backwards and forwards with it will help to clean out dirt. When this has been done, a dressing of archangel tar is applied between the toes.

A more elaborate form of treatment is popular in County Leitrim and County Longford and is quite effective. The ingredients were one pint of hydrogen peroxide 20% and one pint of 40% solution of formalin. The feet were first washed thoroughly with cold water. The hydrogen peroxide is then added until all the fizzing has stopped. The treatment is completed by adding the formalin to the infected area.

A real folk cure for infected feet in cattle is to dress the foot with a preparation of bluestone (copper sulphate). The bluestone is ground very fine, mixed with lard and applied as an ointment.

WARBLE FLY

The swellings on the back under the skin caused by the warble fly were once quite common. The hair around the swelling was clipped carefully and an incision was made through it. The abscess was then opened and cleaned out. The wound was then treated with a diluted solution of Jeyes' Fluid or with salt. Another dressing was white of an egg.

BLACK LEG

There were two methods of treating black leg. One was to make a small incision in the skin and put a clove of garlic inside. The wound was then closed with a stitch, leaving the garlic inside. The other method was to put a red thread through the dewlap and tie the two ends loosely, leaving the thread in position. I am unable to suggest the reason why either of these methods became established, but, as in the case of the red cloth on the cow's tail, the intention may be to drive out evil spirits.

RINGWORM

This is a common disease in all domestic animals but is more often seen in cattle, probably due to the use of a scratching post by which the disease spreads. There are probably many cures, as in the case of human ringworm. I have used three forms of treatment, all of which appear to be effective. The patches may be scrubbed with paraffin oil using a small nail brush. They may be painted with strong tincture of iodine, or they may be painted with archangel tar.

PROLAPSE OF THE UTERUS

This may occur after a difficult delivery in a cow. The prolapsed uterus is cleaned with soft water and manually replaced, but the problem is to prevent the prolapse recurring. A County Leitrim method of doing this was to make a wide belt of strong sacking which went loosely under the belly and across the back of the cow. A stick was placed under the belt of sacking and used to twist the belt as tightly as possible. This prevented the cow from pressing to prolapse the uterus again. Another method was to pass a nail used for shoeing a horse through both labia of the vagina and tie it in position. The pain of the nail would also prevent the cow from pressing.

WORMS

In cattle, worms were treated with a mixture of equal parts of turf, soot and salt. This was made into a paste with water and about a pound of the mixture was given to the cow.

SCOUR

This is very common in cattle and does not always need treatment. If the animal is given large quantities of water and no food the condition will almost always clear up quickly. The only form of treatment I have seen used is boiled comfrey leaves which are broken up and given with a bran mash.

CASSIDY'S RAG

In County Fermanagh, and to a lesser extent in the adjoining counties, a sick animal was treated with Cassidy's rag. When an animal was seen to be sick, someone was sent to a neighbour called Cassidy to ask for a piece of cloth from his clothes. This was put in water which was given to the animal to drink. It is easy to understand why this practice arose. Between the years 1300 and 1600, the Cassidy family were famous physicians to the Maguire chiefs of Fermanagh and on into the eighteenth century the family continued to practice medicine. The use of Cassidy's rag is an echo of the fame of the family. Thirty years ago this practice was well known but some months ago I had difficulty in finding one man who remembered it.

THE CONACH WORM

During the seventeenth century there was a widespread belief that what was called the conach worm was a great cause of disease in cattle. Stories of this worm got to London and about the year 1685 the Royal Society in London wrote to the Dublin Philosophical Society asking for details of the 'Connought worm'. In answer to the enquiry the Secretary, Thomas Molyneaux, sent a drawing of the worm and a description of it which enabled the editor of the Philosophical Transactions to identify it as the caterpillar of the elephant hawk moth. Molyneaux explained that it was generally believed in Ireland that if the worm was eaten by cattle or swine it caused wasting and death. He gave details of the treatment used by the English in Ireland and of that used by the Irish. He ended his letter by saying that the worm had become very rare and in any case he did not believe that the worm did any harm to cattle.

K'eogh mentions this worm. This is what he wrote:

> Murrain Worm. Hib. Chonagh. Lat. Vermis Pecori Noxius Aut Pesteferus. I cannot find any medicinal virtue in this worm: the country people report that it is very pernicious to cattle.

This belief continued on to the middle of the nineteenth century, if not later. John Windle found it in Cork and showed a picture of an amulet in the shape of the worm which was used to protect cattle.

Dineen has an interesting note on the word 'conach'. He says:

> Conach. The elephant hawk moth. Found in dark places and regarded with aversion. On being discovered it is instantly killed as it is believed to sting cattle severely on the muzzle. The ass is supposed to kill it.

CHAPTER III

Diseases of Other Domestic Animals

SHEEP

Sheep suffered from a number of diseases and it was well known that some land was not suitable for them. Everybody knew that they did much better on hard dry land than on soft wet land. One of the most common diseases in sheep was infestation with liver fluke. This was a flat leaf-like worm which has a complicated life history and is found in the liver ducts of the sheep. When heavily infested the animals will not thrive and might even die.

As might be expected, any disease in which the liver was involved was treated with yellow things—iris flowers or yellow wall flowers were used and also the yellow head of the ragwort. None of these methods had any influence on the condition and people generally realised this and I have heard them dismissed as pistrogues. However, when carbon tetra chloride became available, some people realised that it was an effective remedy. One intelligent man I knew used buy it in very large quantities and dispense it to neighbouring sheep farmers.

Foot rot was a common disease of sheep in County Leitrim. The horn of the trotter became soft and the skin between the toes cracked and became severely infected. It was routine to examine the feet at the end of the winter and at the end of the summer. The condition was treated by carefully paring away the soft horn and cleaning out any grossly infected area on the feet. The feet were then painted with archangel tar. Another method was to have the sheep stand in a bath of 10% solution of formalin. The most efficient method of treating foot rot was to use a solution of butter of antimony. This was very painful and people were reluctant to use it because its caustic action might do worse damage to the feet, but used carefully it was quite effective. Butter of antimony has a modern look about it, but it was used as an escharotic early in the eighteenth century.

Treating a sheep infected with maggots is an unpleasant experience. It was most liable to occur in a warm wet July or August. Flies laid eggs in the wool and the larvae when hatched out could very quickly destroy a large area of the skin and, if neglected, an ulcer might form which could cause the death of the animal. The treatment was to clip all the wool around the area of infestation and remove the larvae with the wool. The area was treated with a mixture of buttermilk and salt. Another method was to soak the entire area in Jeyes' Fluid.

PIGS

In a nineteenth century manuscript in the Royal Irish Academy an entry is headed:

> A safe cure for scour in young pigs. Boil flour in milk and add a teaspoonful of alum. Give once a day. Effects a cure.

In County Leitrim swine fever is treated by boiling comfrey roots in milk and adding the entire preparation—roots and milk—to the pig's food. It is necessary to continue this treatment for some weeks.

Pigs gain weight rapidly and unless their diet contains adequate amounts of calcium and vitamin D the bones of their legs will not be able to bear their increasing weight. I have known this condition to have been treated with cod liver oil and lime water added to the feed.

UMBILICAL HERNIA

I have been told that umbilical hernia is not uncommon in pigs and once I had a chance to help with an operation to repair one. A well-grown sucking pig was laid on its back on a table in the open air and held by two people. The operator, despite the squealing of the pig, took great care to ensure that there was no bowel in the sac and then held it firmly closed with both his hands. When he was satisfied that it was safe, he told his assistant, me, to put two large stitches through the sac and tie them firmly on the skin. I managed to do this to his satisfaction. The needle used was about six inches long, slightly curved and flattened at the point and with cutting edges for the first inch or so and the suture material was strong fine cord. Unfortunately I never learned what was the result of the operation.

In County Leitrim and County Clare, the leaves of dandelion and part of the root were boiled and fed to both pigs and poultry, mixed with maze meal.

DOGS

There was little folk medicine used in the care of dogs. If dogs were valuable—gun dogs, or greyhounds, for example —an official veterinary surgeon was called but otherwise little care was taken. It was believed that if a dog ate something harmful he would immediately find and eat scutch grass which made him vomit whatever he had eaten. There was another belief that if one fed too much meat to a dog he was liable to get distemper.

The only diseases of dogs which folk medicine dealt with were diseases of the skin.

Mange, as in horses, was treated with a mixture of trainoil and sulphur. There was a dark ointment which a lady in County Meath made up which was used for skin diseases in dogs, horses and people. I never learned the formula, but from its results it must have been a mercury ointment and probably the one known officially as amoniated mercury ointment.

On a piece of paper which was kept carefully I found a prescription for a lotion to treat mange in dogs. It consisted of:

Black Sulphur	$\frac{1}{4}$ lb.
Turpentine	$1\frac{1}{2}$ oz.
Spirits of Tar	$\frac{1}{2}$ oz.
Mercury ointment	1 oz.
Linseed oil	1 pint

Ringworm in dogs was treated with strong tincture of iodine.

Index